Kids with Celiac Disease

A Family Guide to Raising Happy, Healthy, Gluten-Free Children

Danna Korn

WOODBINE HOUSE 2001

Library of Congress Cataloging-in-Publication Data

Korn, Danna.
   Kids with celiac disease : a family guide to raising happy, healthy, gluten-free children / by Danna Korn.—1st ed.
       p. cm.
   Includes index.
   ISBN 1-890627-21-6 (pbk.)
    1. Celiac disease—Diet therapy. 2. Gluten-free diet. 3. Children—Diseases—Treatment. I. Title.

RJ456.C44 K67 2001
618.92'3995—dc21   00-065022

Manufactured in the United States of America

First edition
10   9   8   7   6   5   4   3   2   1

Dedication

This book is dedicated to those who inspire positive attitudes, even in the face of adversity.

"You can complain because roses have thorns, or you can rejoice because thorns have roses."

—*Ziggy*

"When I hear somebody sigh, 'Life is hard,' I am always tempted to ask, 'Compared to what?'"

—*Sydney Harris*

"Life consists not in holding good cards but in playing those you hold well."

—*Josh Billings*

"Destiny is not a matter of chance, it is a matter of choice; it is not a thing to be waited for, it is a thing to be achieved."

—*William Jennings Bryan*

"The problem is not that there are problems. The problem is expecting otherwise and thinking that having problems is a problem."

—*Theodore Rubin*

While there is really no need to explain the relevance of these analogies to those of us who are raising celiac kids, I hope everyone who reads this book will make the connection and guide their children toward an optimistic, productive, gluten-free future.

"I've decided that after air, water, and dirt, the next most common substance on the planet must be gluten." :-)
        —Toni Nolte, Overland Park, Kansas

Table of Contents

Advisory Board

Margaret V. Austin, Ph.D.
Clinical psychologist
Carlsbad, CA

Sandro Drago, Master Scientist
Visiting Scientist
University of Maryland, Baltimore

Nancy Patin Falini, M.A., R.D.
Dietitian specializing in celiac disease
West Chester, PA

Alessio Fasano, M.D.
Professor of Pediatrics, Medicine, and Physiology
University of Maryland School of Medicine
Baltimore, MD

Tania Gerarduzzi, M.D.
University of Trieste, Italy
Postdoctoral fellow,
University of Maryland, Baltimore

Peter H.R. Green, M.D.
Clinical Professor of Medicine
Columbia University College of Physicians and Surgeons
New York, NY

Elaine Monarch
Founder/Executive Director, Celiac Disease Foundation
Studio City, CA

Thomas W. Self, M.D., FAAP
Pediatric gastroenterologist
Professor of Clinical Pediatrics
University of California, San Diego

Acknowledgements

I believe I speak for the vast number of people who have or know people who have celiac disease when I say I am deeply grateful to the many experts who have researched the subject of celiac disease and shared their information through printed material and/or the Internet.

I'd like to thank my Advisory Board members for their support, encouragement, and suggestions: Tom Self, M.D.; Elaine Monarch, Founder/Executive Director, Celiac Disease Foundation; Nancy Patin Falini, M.A., R.D.; Margaret V. Austin, Ph.D.; Alessio Fasano, M.D.; Tania Gerarduzzi, M.D.; and Sandro Drago.

And I suppose it goes without saying (but while I'm on a roll...) that acknowledgement and gratitude go to my family members for their support and understanding when I needed quiet time to write this book— and of course to our son, Tyler, and to every child with celiac disease, because they have been the inspiration and motivation for the time and energy that we've devoted to helping other families—an effort that brings us endless fulfillment and gratification.

A Word about Terminology

This book is intended to be useful to parents of children who have any dietary restrictions, but in particular, we focus on gluten intolerance (an inability to eat foods containing gluten). This includes children who have been diagnosed with:

- celiac disease,
- gluten-sensitive enteropathy (GSE), and
- nontropical sprue,

which are all just different names for the same disorder.

It also includes children with dermatitis herpetiformis, a disorder closely related to celiac disease, and other children who cannot eat gluten due to allergies, personal preferences, or other reasons.

Most of the information in this book applies equally to all children with any condition calling for a gluten-free diet. To simplify matters, however, we refer primarily to celiac disease (spelled "coeliac" in Europe) throughout the book.

Foreword

Rich & Shelley Gannon

"KIDS WITH CELIAC DISEASE offers a refreshing, positive approach to dealing with the challenges of raising a child with severe dietary restrictions, and has practical suggestions for any situation that families raising children with celiac disease might encounter."

We can empathize with the parents of children who have severe dietary restrictions, because after a long, mysterious illness, our daughter, Danielle, was diagnosed with celiac disease in 1999. At first it was overwhelming. Other than our gastroenterologist and a distant support group for adults, we felt all alone. We had so many questions, fears, and concerns about the future.

Our biggest concern was to make sure Danielle was happy and healthy. One of the most exasperating elements to all of this was that there was no single source of information that we could turn to day in and day out, no matter where we were or what time it was. Finding *any* information on celiac disease was difficult, but what we really wanted was a "manual"— something that addressed the emotions we were dealing with as well as the practical questions we had about her new gluten-free diet. We needed a guide for ourselves, and for our family and friends, that would tell us all how to deal with our daughter's new lifestyle in a positive, healthy manner.

Kids with Celiac Disease is a godsend for our family and other families raising children with celiac disease. It answered all of our questions, and many that we didn't even know we had. As Danielle grows, we know we will face new and difficult challenges . . . and it's reassuring to know that we'll have this book to refer to.

Kids with Celiac Disease offers a refreshing, positive approach to dealing with the challenges of raising a child with severe dietary restrictions, and has practical suggestions for any situation that families raising children with celiac disease might encounter. We found it to be witty, easy to read, and most of all, comforting.

We would like to say "thank you," Danna, for taking the time to write this book. It is going to help so many families and raise much-needed awareness!

Rich Gannon is the quarterback for the Oakland Raiders football team. His wife, Shelley, was an All-American gymnast at the University of Minnesota, and is now a full-time mother to their two daughters, Alexis and Danielle.

Preface

This Book: What It Is and What It Isn't

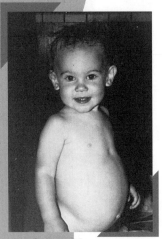

October 1990
By the time he was 15 months old, Tyler looked malnourished. Doctors were still telling us there was nothing wrong with him.

Since you're reading this book, you probably have or know a child diagnosed with or suspected of having celiac disease. Adapting to the diagnosis means an entirely new lifestyle that encompasses much more than "simply" a dietary change. It's huge. It means you'll have to think before driving through a fast food restaurant; you'll need to make special accommodations for birthday parties and outings; you'll need to educate just about everyone who ever comes in contact with your child. And, at least at first, it will seem as though there is *nothing* your child can eat. He can't even lick an envelope! If the news is still fresh, and, perhaps, even if it isn't, you're most likely experiencing a myriad of emotions, ranging from panic to hysteria, confusion, and relief.

I know you want to skip to the end where I tell you the magic key to making it all easier, but reading these preliminaries may actually be worthwhile. If nothing else, you will find out that my family and I can empathize. We have a child with celiac disease, so we know what you're going through. We sincerely hope that this book will simplify your life, help you deal with day-to-day situations, show you how to provide the most supportive emotional environment for your child, give you an optimistic outlook on your child's future, and comfort you when you feel that no one understands. Oh—and by the way—it really *does* get easier.

Why I Wrote This Book

Our son was diagnosed with celiac disease when he was eighteen months old. Prior to the diagnosis, we had the same story most of you have had: a child with twenty diarrhea diapers a day; huge, distended belly, skinny arms, lack of energy; and visits to several insensitive doctors who had no idea what was *really* wrong, but had the gall to tell us, with that condescending, why-are-you-wasting-my-time-I-have-real-patients-waiting tone, that there was nothing wrong with our child. One pediatrician actually took my hand, and with a kind, but patronizing smile, said, "I know, honey. Mommies get really neurotic about diarrhea. It won't last forever, you know." But of course—why hadn't I realized that it was *my* neurosis that was resulting in the twenty diarrhea diapers a day?

Nine months and three doctors later, I was still apparently neurotic. When our insurance changed and we were forced to go to a new pediatric group, I thought nothing of dragging in a listless, lethargic baby with skinny arms and legs and a belly that begged for jokes about a pregnant baby. By then my husband and I had accepted the fact that we must have just gotten one of those kids who poops a lot, and I sure wasn't going to talk about it any further, for fear *everyone* would then know how neurotic I had actually been. So when, during a routine ear check, the new pediatrician expressed concern about Tyler's distended belly, I broke down and cried, thankful that finally someone was going to believe that there really *was* something wrong with my son.

You can probably guess what we went through next. Daily visits to the hospital, working with the pediatric gastroenterologist to rule out everything from cystic fibrosis to cancer to a rare blood disorder. A week later, when he suggested that we do a biopsy and check for yet another disease we had never heard of—celiac disease—we numbly nodded our approval and signed yet another release form. Several months and three biopsies later, we had our confirmation. The good news was that there was a label for what was wrong with our son. The bad news was that it was going to require more than a few changes in our lives. A bittersweet diagnosis, indeed.

Our Son's Diagnosis — What Now?

For the first three days after Tyler was diagnosed with celiac disease, he ate nothing but french fries and Fritos. We were scared to death we were going to poison him. I got brave and decided to head to my local grocery store—after all, I'm an intelligent person—how hard could it be to read a few labels? Two hours later, I left with tear-stained cheeks and four bags of Fritos.

Thinking quickly and pulling myself together, I headed to the local health food store. Thankfully, they actually carried frozen loaves of gluten-free bread! I choked at the nearly $5 per-loaf price tag, but remembering it was for my baby boy, I cheerfully bought five loaves and headed home with a renewed sense of optimism.

I covered a piece of toast with jelly and nearly cried with joy as I handed it to him. Well, almost handed it to him. Because, as any of you who have bought that stuff know, when you look at it too hard, it falls apart. So I gathered the pieces, "glued" them together with the jelly, and held my breath while I watched him take his first bite of gluten-free bread. He spit that piece of bread so far I was finding pieces of it three days later! Obviously, I was going to have to work on finding some better foods, or even—gasp—make my own!

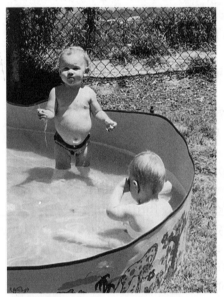

July 1991
Tyler had been on a gluten-free diet for two months and was showing signs of improvement.

My husband and I realized that what we needed was a little support. So we asked our pediatric gastroenterologist where we could find the local support group for parents of kids with celiac disease. You know this next part: "The what?" There was no such group. There *was*, however, a group for adults with celiac disease, and we figured that was just as good.

Still somewhat in shock from the diagnosis, off we went to our first celiac support group. We expected to be greeted with pamphlets and flyers on how to deal with babysitters and other caretakers, going to school, and Halloween and other special occasions.

Please don't misunderstand me here. Those groups are *great*, and I so very much appreciate their hard work. But, while the group we met seemed friendly and knowledgeable, we quickly tired of hearing about which fat-free foods were gluten-free, which senior supplements were gluten-free (the average age of the group was nearly double my own), which Thai restaurants were safe (oh sure, our two-year-old was begging for Thai), and how to prevent weight gain once on a gluten-free diet. It became clear that adults with celiac disease had different concerns than I had. I wanted *real* information I could actually use, and I was growing impatient with the lack of pertinent, helpful advice on raising *kids* with celiac disease.

I figured maybe it was the *previous* meeting when all of the parental advice had been given, and I had just missed out. Maybe if I asked the right questions....

So, at the end of the meeting, I eagerly stood up and explained that my baby boy had just been diagnosed, and wondered where I could find the pamphlets on raising kids with celiac disease. Not a word. After an awkward silence, the room began to buzz again with talk of more adult issues, and my husband and I realized we were completely alone in our plight. (Thankfully, a lot has changed in the last several years, and these local support groups are now actually quite knowledgeable about raising kids with celiac disease!)

R.O.C.K. (Raising Our Celiac Kids) Was Born

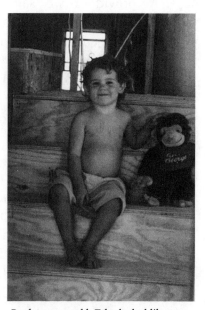

By three years old, Tyler looked like any other three-year-old child.

It was then, in 1991, that we decided that once we got a handle on things, we'd be there to help other people. So we decided to start a support group for families of kids with celiac disease. We came up with the name R.O.C.K., which stands for Raising Our Celiac Kids, and set out to find people who might want to be included in our group. We contacted our pediatric gastroenterologist, figuring he probably had dozens of families looking for support in raising their celiac kids. He put us in touch with *the* other family that he knew of in San Diego County. With some local publicity and networking with other pediatricians, slowly our membership grew to include several families.

Today, R.O.C.K. is an international support group, and we answer questions from families around the world. The calls we get from parents of newly diagnosed children are the most satisfying. In the beginning, we can hear the fear, the frustration, the panic, and the desperation. And we recognize it because we were there. But by the end of the conversation, they tell us they're relieved, and they know that they can move on.

What This Book Isn't . . .

It isn't a product guide. In fact, there will be little mention of specific brand names. If we do refer to a commercially sold product or food item, you should always check its status to confirm that it is, in fact, gluten-free.

This book isn't a cookbook. It isn't a medical guide, and it most definitely is not a panacea for all of the difficult situations you may encounter in raising your child.

What This book Is . . .

Because we remember how desperate we were for menu and snack suggestions, we have included plenty of ideas that will keep your child well fed for days. We provide lists of safe and forbidden ingredients, and everything else you will need to know to raise a celiac child. There are, by the way, several good product guides, cookbooks, and other resources listed in the Resource Guide at the end of this book.

You may want to give this book to your family, teachers, friends, and people with whom your child spends a lot of time. It's a family survival guide!

But more than that, this book is intended to help you deal with the unique situations we face as parents of celiac kids:

- What exactly is gluten?
- How do I prepare my child for the testing?
- How do I find out what foods are okay for him?
- How do we send him to school without worrying?
- What can I feed him for quick snacks?
- What do we do for Halloween and other treat-oriented holidays?
- How do we explain this to babysitters, day care people, and other caretakers?
- Why am I so angry?
- What do we do for birthday parties?
- How do I handle the well-meaning-but-cookie-slipping friends?
- My family is in denial—how do we explain this to them?
- Can we ever go out to dinner?
- How do you travel?
- Can I send him to camp?
- What do I do when he cheats on his diet and intentionally eats gluten?
- What should we do if he accidentally gets gluten?
- Will he suffer from teasing and peer pressure?

- How do I help him handle this emotionally so he can be "just a kid?"
- Why doesn't my doctor understand?
- Will he outgrow this?
- What other conditions are associated with celiac disease?
- Can I ever shop at a "regular" grocery store again?
- Does the whole family need to be gluten-free?
- How healthy is the gluten-free diet?

These are things that most adults with celiac disease don't talk about in their support groups and things that *other* parents never need to give a second thought to. Things that consume us, frustrate us, and cause us to feel anger, guilt, and sadness. They are, however, most definitely things that we can learn to deal with. This book will remind you that you're not alone, and that it does get easier. It's a compilation of lessons we've learned, most of them the hard way, and advice we've gathered from other families raising kids with celiac disease. We hope that you will find it helpful in raising a happy, healthy gluten-free kid.

Introduction

Thomas W. Self, M.D., FAAP

> *"The rapid, almost miraculous, recovery in children with celiac disease who follow a strict gluten-free diet is one of the major rewards for the treating physician, as well as for the patient and parents. After months and often years of poor health, the parents see their sickly child blossom into good health and robust activity."*

Every physician carries within himself a clinical danger list, so to speak, of diseases that are often misdiagnosed or undiagnosed for long periods of time, resulting in patients who grow sicker and sicker without the proper treatment.

For me, as a pediatric gastroenterologist, the condition that is always at the top of my personal checklist of illnesses to exclude is celiac disease. This disease, when undiagnosed, can insidiously debilitate a young child, leading to little or no weight gain, extreme lethargy, delays in reaching developmental milestones, and severe growth failure. Unfortunately, however, many American physicians overlook celiac disease as a possible diagnosis, because most medical schools in this country teach that the disease is rare. This is especially unfortunate since a relatively uncomplicated treatment program (a gluten-free diet for life) produces a rapid improvement of symptoms and a dramatic return to health.

Although we now know celiac disease to be caused by an abnormal immune reaction to gluten that occurs in genetically predisposed individuals, this knowledge is only recent. For centuries, after celiac symptoms were first described around the first century

A.D., physicians had no clue as to why the disease occurred and could only watch helplessly as their patients wasted away.

A major breakthrough in the understanding of the cause of celiac disease came during the German occupation of Holland during World War II. The German troops commandeered the protein-rich grains, wheat, rye, and barley, leaving the Dutch population to exist on potato and rice starch. Children who had suffered from celiac symptoms before the war recovered and thrived on the new dietary regimen, only to relapse when they resumed eating wheat products after the war ended. W.K. Dicke, a pediatrician in Holland, was the first to make the connection between celiac disease and the ingestion of foods containing gluten. Thereafter, for the first time, a gluten-free diet became the keystone for the treatment of celiac disease. Shortly afterwards, in the early 1950s, researchers were first able to biopsy the small intestine and study where the damage occurs in celiac disease, as well as observe the dramatic cellular changes that occur in this disease.

Over the past thirty years or so, research into the causes of celiac disease has continued to reveal much more about how and why the disease occurs and why certain populations are at greater risk. Researchers have also identified certain other diseases and conditions closely associated with celiac disease, including thyroiditis, rheumatoid arthritis, liver disease, Down syndrome, and dermatitis herpetiformis.

Despite this growing body of knowledge and the fact that the incidence of celiac disease is now estimated to be as high as 1 in 150 people, it still remains one of the most under-diagnosed diseases. This is largely because, until recently, diagnosis was based entirely on the presence of the "classic symptoms": diarrhea, weight loss, and abdominal distention occurring shortly after the introduction of gluten-containing foods into the diet of infants or young children. Many physicians are unaware that celiac disease can present with other symptoms, including constipation, arthritis, and early-onset diabetes, and that it can first appear in adolescence or even in adulthood. Furthermore, managed care, with its emphasis on limiting testing on patients, can cause delays in diagnosis until the patient's condition becomes more chronic or severe.

In my clinical experience, most children with celiac disease have been evaluated by at least two, and sometimes three or more, physicians before coming to my practice. Some of their symptoms may differ from the classic symptoms outlined above, but many of them also have marked diarrhea, abdominal distention, and lethargy when I first see them. Their parents are usually understandably anxious about their child's illness. In addition, mixed with that worry is often a concern that I will not take them and their complaints seriously and they will be forced, yet again, to seek out the medical help that they need.

One of the sickest children I was ever asked to evaluate was a two-year-old boy with severely delayed growth, wasted arms and legs, and an enormously distended abdomen. His parents had been accused of possible child abuse, even though they had taken their son to two different doctors who could not identify a medical reason for his condition. The child was brought to me for still another evaluation only when it became apparent that his symptoms did not clear up under the supervision of state workers, with the child being fed a "regular" diet. A small bowel biopsy revealed that the villi in his intestine were flattened, indicating damage from gluten intolerance. A gluten-free diet rapidly resolved the boy's symptoms, and he was returned to his relieved parents—a dramatic, if somewhat unusual, presentation of celiac disease!

The rapid, almost miraculous, recovery in children with celiac disease who follow a strict gluten-free diet is one of the major rewards for the treating physician, as well as for the patient and parents. After months and often years of poor health, the parents see their sickly child blossom into good health and robust activity.

Sometimes, it can be difficult to convince parents of the need to put their child on a gluten-free diet. Usually, they express initial disbelief and frustration over the diagnosis, especially if the symptoms have been present for a long period. I explain that a protein complex called gluten cannot be properly assimilated by their child and actually acts as a toxin whenever ingested. I emphasize the vital importance of remaining on the gluten-free diet for life, even at my very first meeting with parents after the diagnosis. I feel it is important to avoid the term "allergy" in explaining celiac disease to parents, since, in my experience, this term tends to demean both the critical significance of the diagnosis, and dilute the importance of following the dietary restrictions—*without exception*—for life. Celiac disease is not hay fever and should not be regarded as such! Equally important for parents to understand, however, is that celiac disease is completely treatable: Children with the disease can live normally and enjoy good health as long as they stay on a gluten-free diet.

Health providers, as well as parents, should leap at the chance to avail themselves of the accurate and current information provided in this book. **Kids with Celiac Disease** should go a long way toward increasing awareness of the existence and prevalence of this devastating, but completely treatable illness. And since it is written by an author who is pulling from her own well of experience as a mother of a child with celiac disease, it should also reassure parents that putting a child on a gluten-free diet does not spell the end of normal family life. I can only hope that readers of this book will be able to avoid the agony and frustration experienced by countless children and their parents who did not have such a user-friendly guide at their disposal.

What It's Like to Be a Kid with Celiac Disease

Tyler Korn

Hello, my name is Tyler Korn. I'm eleven years old, and I wanted to talk about my experience with celiac disease.

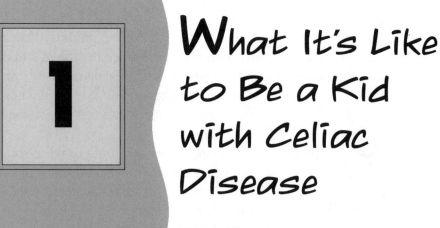

When I was little, we didn't know what was wrong with me, but my parents knew I was really sick. Back then I was just eating regular food like you guys, and I would start getting sick. I don't remember it now, but my parents say that I was so sick they were scared I might even die. They took me to a bunch of doctors, and no one could figure out what was wrong. Finally we met a doctor who realized I was very sick, and he sent us to another doctor who figured out I had celiac disease.

Having celiac disease doesn't bother me. My friends all understand, and some of them even say they want *their* hamburgers without buns, or their ice cream in a bowl instead of a cone.

We make a lot of our own breads and cookies and things, and I do a lot of cooking myself!

Really, it's not something I think about very often. I'm busy with baseball, motocross, and other sports, and it seems like those are the things I think about. My parents ask me sometimes what it feels like to have celiac disease, but it really

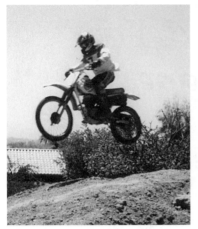

doesn't feel like anything. It's really not that big of a deal. Maybe it used to be for them, but it isn't for me.

My parents asked me to write some advice for you parents who have kids with celiac disease. I guess my advice is: Don't freak out. It's probably really confusing and scary at first—I don't know, because I don't remember that part of it. But these days, it's just no big deal. I hope that makes you feel better . . . to know that we kids with celiac disease can lead perfectly normal lives.

The other advice I'd give is to let your kids be in control. I read my own labels and make all of my own food decisions. Sometimes my parents get scared that I'm going to make mistakes, but I know what I'm doing. (I am almost a man!) Sometimes I do make a mistake, and I get a really bad stomachache—worse than the flu. It feels like a sharp pain in my stomach, and sometimes it makes me tired and lazy. But it goes away, and then I know not to eat that food again!

I hope you all enjoy this book, and I hope it makes it easier for you and your family to deal with celiac disease.

Good luck!

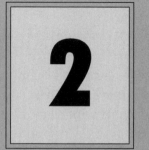

2

What Is Celiac Disease?

(and nontropical sprue, dermatitis herpetiformis, gluten-sensitive enteropathy, and general gluten intolerance)

What Is Celiac Disease?

Celiac disease is a genetic disorder in which gluten intolerance leads to damage to the lining of the small intestine. In other words, people with celiac disease have a sensitivity to *gluten*—a protein found in wheat, rye, oats, and barley (as well as malt, which is made from barley).

In people with celiac disease, gluten damages the *villi* in the small intestine. Villi are the small hair-like projections that are responsible for absorbing nutrients from digested food (see illustration at left). Eventually, the villi may become partially or even completely flattened, and unable to do their job. When this happens, the body is deprived of basic nutrients, and the person may become

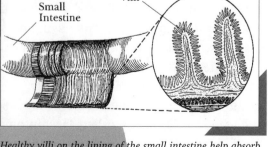

Healthy villi on the lining of the small intestine help absorb nutrients.

malnourished and dehydrated. There *is* good news, however. The damage is completely reversible if gluten is removed from the diet.

What Is Gluten, Anyway?

Gluten is the protein portion of wheat, rye, barley, and oats. (Their botanical names are, respectively, triticum, secale, hordeum, and avena.) There is actually a controversy over whether or not oats are toxic to people with celiac disease; to simplify matters, we will refer to oats as one of the forbidden grains. Related gluten-containing grains include triticale, kamut, spelt, semolina, and durum. Gluten is also a common food additive. Because gluten is high in protein, some manufacturers add it to their food products to increase the protein content. Gluten is what makes breads stick together, which is why gluten-free breads sometimes fall apart.

To get a little more technical, there are actually two classifications of protein: the prolamines and the glutelins. The prolamine in gluten is called gliadin, which is the real culprit in celiac disease. Prolamine (also spelled prolamin) is the alcohol-soluble part of protein, so gliadin is the alcohol-soluble fraction of wheat.

Each grain has a different amount of prolamine, or gliadin. The amount of gliadin is what determines the type of reaction from someone with celiac disease. The reason your child with celiac disease has different levels of reactions to different foods is partially due to the varying amounts of prolamines in different grains.

What Are the Symptoms of Celiac Disease?

The symptoms of celiac disease result from the inability of the small intestine to absorb nutrients from food as it is digested. These symptoms may appear as soon as your child begins to eat gluten—usually just before her first birthday—or they may not show up until later. Interestingly, the two most common age ranges for exhibiting celiac symptoms are the toddler years (1-4) and the 50s. (See Chapter 21 for information on possible "triggers" of celiac disease.)

Celiac disease is difficult to diagnose because the symptoms are so varied. Some people exhibit "classic" symptoms such as diarrhea, malabsorption, gas, and bloating. Others may experience fatigue, anemia, irritability, vomiting, short stature, or difficulty concentrating.

It is extremely important to note that some people with celiac disease show absolutely no symptoms whatsoever. These are called "asymptomatic" or "silent" celiacs, but the damage is still being done! It is also important to realize that just because your child does *not* show these "classic" symptoms does *not* mean she does not have celiac disease. Celiac disease is a diagnosis based on the abnormality in the intestines, not the symptoms.

"Classic" and Common Symptoms for Infants and Toddlers

- Diarrhea—oftentimes the diarrhea is described by parents as being particularly foul smelling and foamy in appearance.
- Failure to thrive (below average weight gain or increase in height)
- Projectile vomiting
- Distended abdomen
- Lack of muscle definition (throughout the body)
- Dental disorders (ridges and changes in pigmentation in secondary teeth)
- Irritability
- Listlessness
- Lack of desire to eat
- Low levels of calcium, vitamin B12, and folic acid
- Extreme separation anxiety or excessive dependence on parents (probably because they're in pain and get comfort from parents)

"Classic" and Common Symptoms for Children and Adults

- Gastrointestinal distress (cramping, bloating, gas)
- Diarrhea
- Constipation
- Steatorrhea (foul, frothy, sometimes floating stools)
- Anemia and/or nutritional deficiencies
- Lack of muscle definition
- Delayed onset of puberty
- Weight loss
- Lack of desire to eat
- Emotional disturbances including irritability, depression, difficulty concentrating, and excessive dependence

If left untreated, celiac disease can cause a number of long-term and even life-threatening conditions, including:

- Osteoporosis and other bone disease, such as osteomalacia, osteoperia, and rickets
- Bone "pain"
- Weight loss
- Epilepsy
- Internal hemorrhaging
- Central and peripheral nervous system disorders

- Pancreatic disease or disorders
- Intestinal lymphoma (cancer)
- Anemia
- Chronic diarrhea
- Lactose intolerance
- Lack of dental enamel formation (in children)
- Infertility (in both men and women)
- In women, miscarriage, delayed start of menstruation, premature menopause
- A variety of emotional disturbances, including chronic fatigue, irritability, an inability to concentrate, Attention Deficit Disorder (ADD/ADHD)-type symptoms (such as hyperactivity, impulsivity), and even schizophrenic behavior.

Could My Child Just Have "a Touch" of Celiac Disease?

There is no such thing as having "a touch of celiac disease." Some people may have "milder" symptoms, or even no symptoms at all, but the damage is still being done internally. The reason some people show fewer or no symptoms ("asymptomatic" or "compensated-latent disease") is because: 1) the length of the small bowel that has been damaged is shorter, or 2) there is less damage to the mucous membrane, or the lining, of the small intestine.

In celiac disease, the damage starts in the small intestine just beyond the stomach, and works its way down (see illustration at right). If the damage is only near the stomach, there are several feet of small intestine left to compensate for the damaged portion that does not absorb food and nutrients. That remaining portion can absorb enough of the food and liquid that the person may not ever have diarrhea and other classic symptoms. It's important to note, however, that even though there are no classic symptoms, gluten is al-

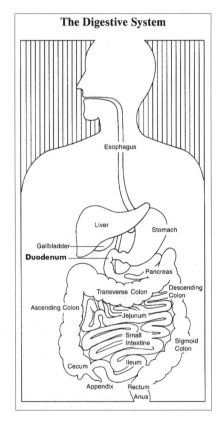

The Digestive System

The damage in celiac disease starts in the duodenum, the area of the small intestine that connects with the stomach.

ways damaging to people with celiac disease. No matter how slight the damage may be, it can—and generally will—spread. In addition, because the upper part of the intestine is where iron, folic acid, calcium, and fat soluble vitamins (K, A, D, E) are absorbed, everyone with celiac disease is at risk of malnutrition.

How Common Is Celiac Disease?

You may think celiac disease is rare, but it's not! Worldwide, celiac disease is thought to occur in approximately one in 150 to one in 250 people. It is most common in people of European descent, and apparently affects females about three times more often than males.

At one time it was thought that celiac disease was very rare in people of African and Asian descent, but recent studies indicate otherwise. It also occurs in other races, including North Africans, Arabs, and Slavic people. There are a variety of theories as to why celiac disease now seems more common in non-Europeans than previously. Perhaps at one time the incidence *was* lower due to a lack of gluten in the diet (i.e., wheat was not the most common grain in their diet), or perhaps cases were missed due to a lack of proper diagnosis. Then again, people in some countries may truly have a lower genetic susceptibility.

What is Dermatitis Herpetiformis?

Dermatitis herpetiformis (DH) is a "sister" to celiac disease. Everyone with DH has celiac disease, but their primary symptoms—a very severe rash on their skin—are external. Internally, gluten usually wreaks the same havoc on the small intestine as it does in people with celiac disease. Seventy to eighty percent of people with DH have coexisting damage in the intestine.

DH is characterized by blistering, intensely itchy skin. Often it is initially misdiagnosed as eczema, but DH does not respond to eczema medications. The rash is found on the elbows, buttocks, knees, back, face, and/or scalp, and is usually symmetrical, meaning that it occurs in a mirror image from left to right. A small percentage (about 5 percent) of people with celiac disease have these skin lesions, as well.

DH is diagnosed by a small skin biopsy taken at the blister site. If IgA (immunoglobulin A) is present (see page 144), it confirms that there has been a reaction to the ingestion of gluten, and DH is the probable diagnosis. The treatment is a strict gluten-free diet.

How Is Celiac Disease Treated?

This is the beauty of celiac disease. After diagnosis, a strict gluten-free diet will be prescribed. Then you can expect your child to improve immediately! Depending upon the severity of the symptoms before diagnosis, you will see a remarkably happier child, who is more content and energetic, and has a better appetite. The bloated belly will slowly disappear, diarrhea should subside within a couple of weeks, and gas, cramping, and general discomfort will be a thing of the past. Growth, if previously affected, will increase quickly.

After a few weeks on the gluten-free diet, most people find that their energy levels increase and that they begin to "feel better" overall. This is because celiac disease, when untreated, prevents absorption of certain nutrients, especially iron, calcium, and folic acid, even when supplements are taken. The malabsorption of iron results in anemia, leading to weakness, lethargy, and an overall feeling of fatigue. Many physicians recommend taking vitamin and mineral supplements, at least for a while after initiating a gluten-free diet, to compensate for the deficiencies that existed before.

Symptoms aside, you can also expect a little (or a lot of) resistance from your child regarding the new diet. That's okay; it's a new concept for everyone. You will most likely be feeling a myriad of emotions yourself, which will be reflected in your child's moods and behavior. Time will heal that, too.

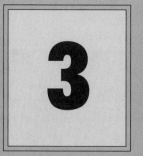

3

Panic, Anger, Grief, Denial,
and Other Emotions You Can Look Forward To

The Bittersweet Diagnosis . . . Then Panic Sets In

Ah, but it's a bittersweet diagnosis, isn't it? After a long ordeal, you're assured that your child will need no medication or surgery, and has a prognosis of perfect health. It's just that at first it seems there's nothing on the planet that you can feed him.

Most likely, you had a difficult time arriving at a diagnosis. It's an all-too-common story. You have a child who is sick and getting sicker, yet doctors can't seem to figure out what's wrong. Often they wave you away with some vague "explanation" of why your child has symptoms, but with no diagnosis and no understanding of how to make your kid feel better.

Those of us who know the symptoms of celiac disease can spot it a mile away, yet most doctors don't think of it, and many even refuse to test for it when it is suggested as a possibility. Doctors and nurses toss out possible explanations for your child's symptoms as though they're reviewing a grocery list: cystic fibrosis, check; blood disease, check; cancer, check. It's impossible to describe the sensations we experience while waiting to find out what's wrong with our babies.

The truth is that we really should be thankful once the diagnosis is made. In many children, the diagnosis is missed, and they suffer their entire lives. Others are misdiagnosed, and gluten continues to wreak havoc on their system, while the blame is erroneously placed on lactose, irritable bowel syndrome, or other conditions.

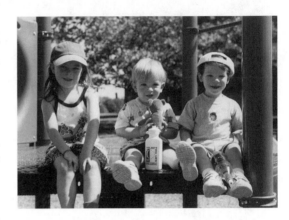

So, if your child has been diagnosed, you're fortunate. I know, it's hard to see beyond the "difficult" diet at first, but it does get easier, and there are many resources available to get you through it. A gluten-free lifestyle is extremely healthy, and there are no medications required, no surgeries, and no long-term difficulties, if a strict gluten-free diet is adhered to.

Panic, Anger, Grief, Denial, and Other Emotions You Can Look Forward To

It's important to know that it's perfectly normal to experience a myriad of emotions when your child has been diagnosed with celiac disease. You're not selfish if you feel self-pity; you're not a "bad parent" if you find yourself angry; you're not alone if you feel an overwhelming sense of grief, and even loss.

"My little girl was just diagnosed a week ago. Someone gave me another mother's phone number and suggested I call, but I'm so overwhelmed with emotion that I'm paralyzed. I can't even think of the questions to ask."
—*Debi B.*

Many parents, while in the chasm of these sometimes-overwhelming emotions, withdraw and are unsure of what to do next. Understanding that these feelings are normal is an important step in overcoming them.

People tend to progress through a series of emotions in response to bad news or a loss. If you think about it, having your child diagnosed with celiac disease is a loss of a kind. Perhaps it is the loss of the image you may have had for your child's future. The specific meaning of this information varies widely among individuals. However, this type of event typically requires that people go through a period of adjustment in order to integrate the new information into their existing mental framework. Below is my take, as a parent, on the adjustment process. For a more formal description of the adjustment process through a psychologist's eyes, see Chapter Twenty-Four.

Panic

Generally, the first emotion you'll experience is *panic*. What on earth will you feed this child? What if you poison him? How do you explain it to your friends and family? There are a number of issues that may be concerning you at this point, and they all must be sorted through before you can move on. It can feel quite overwhelming as implications and concerns begin to arise. However, it's important for you to realize that the panic you feel at first is a normal part of the adaptation process—and it will pass.

Analysis Paralysis

Closely related to panic is "analysis paralysis." People who are more analytically inclined sometimes find that they get so involved in trying to figure out the "whys," "hows," and "what-ifs" that they can think of little else. The problem with this condition is that it's impossible to move forward, and to be a positive role model for your children, friends, and family.

Anger

Unfortunately, panic will most likely give way to other "normal" but unpleasant emotions. There's a blurry line between the initial panic and subsequent anger, but most parents experience anger early on. It's not directed at your child, of course, and it's completely normal. Some people are angry at God or Fate. This may be especially true for parents whose child has another condition such as Down syndrome or cystic fibrosis in addition to celiac disease and can't understand what their child did to deserve this double helping of medical problems. Some parents are angry at the pediatricians who sent them away telling them their child was fine. Many are angry at food manufacturers who won't just make it simple by putting "gluten" on the ingredients list. Some are even angry at whomever passed the "defective gene" to their child.

It's important to recognize your anger as a normal part of adaptation, but also to develop appropriate outlets for it. Some people benefit from having someone to talk to; others feel better if they can write in a journal or have another type of artistic outlet. Still others simply throw themselves actively into the task at hand. Whatever your coping style, be sure to put some effort into taking care of yourself. You will need to be the guiding force for the changes in your child's life.

Remember that your child will likely be angry, too, even if he's too young to understand the diagnosis. He may be angry at you for taking away the foods he enjoys, or angry that he feels deprived. Older children often feel anger at the same people and circumstances that adults experience: anger at the relative who passed the gene; anger at God; anger at food manufacturers.

Help your child deal with anger in an appropriate manner. Let him talk, draw angry pictures, or whatever else helps him feel as though he's being heard. Listen carefully. Tell him you understand, and that he has every right to feel angry. But make sure he understands that you are there to help him, and that together you will learn how to live a happy, healthy gluten-free life.

Some kids feel no anger whatsoever. This too is normal, and should not be considered to be apathy, repression, or any other "abnormal" response.

Grief

Most parents do experience grief with regard to their child's diagnosis. As mentioned above, grief is a very normal response to any perceived loss. You may feel sad because you worry that your child's life won't be absolutely perfect, that he may be teased, or that he may experience health problems.

"Deanna was diagnosed six years ago. At first I felt so sad—sad for her, sad for myself, and sad for the rest of the family. As I learned to handle the diet, I felt better about things. But every couple of years, as she goes through different phases of her life and her diet causes various challenges for her, I find myself feeling sad again. I wonder if it is normal to feel this way, especially so long after the original diagnosis."
—Sarah M.

It is very important to recognize your grief and to allow yourself a grieving period. Difficult emotions tend to become more manageable when dealt with directly than they are when ignored. However, it is also important not to dwell on it. Your own attitude about your child's health will have a significant impact on his attitude about himself. Grief is one of the emotions that may rear its ugly head every couple of years and must be addressed again each time.

Denial

Denial is a common emotion that may occur a few months after your child has been on a gluten-free diet and is doing better. Nearly everyone says that their child starts looking so good, feeling so healthy, that they start to suspect that maybe there was never anything wrong in the first place! Often parents who are "challenging" their child's diet (after the first biopsy and before the second) notice that their child doesn't show any response to gluten. (See page 147.) This is typical, and so is your probable (but overly hopeful and erroneous) conclusion that your child doesn't actually have celiac disease.

Denial often occurs again when your child is older—ten years old or so. Usually the reason it occurs at this stage is because your child may get some gluten, whether accidentally or because he cheated, and will have no response (see information on "Honeymoon Period," page 135). It is common for parents and kids both to eagerly assume the child has "outgrown" the condition, or that he never had it, and was misdiagnosed. Be cautious about jumping to conclusions. Chances are, the diagnosis was correct, and, unfortunately, children *don't* grow out of it.

The danger in this stage is that there's the temptation to cheat—to go ahead and give the child gluten, since he "probably doesn't have celiac disease anyway!" Don't do it. This denial phase too will pass, and reality will set in.

Fear and Heartache

Fear and heartache seem to go hand in hand. Every time your child has a tummy-ache (and all kids get them, remember), you'll wonder if he's gotten some gluten. You may even be afraid that you aren't following the diet closely enough. Try not to become consumed with fear. Deal with it together as a family, and this will help you relax.

The anguish we feel on our kids' behalf may raise questions that can haunt you: Will this make him less appealing as a husband? Will he be traumatized and psychologically impaired? Will his friends make fun of him? Can I handle the sorrow if they do? Can he? If he has another diagnosis such as Down syndrome or epilepsy, will celiac disease affect his ability to live independently as an adult? What will his future bring? Relax. These thoughts disappear as you *and* your child become more comfortable with the diet and realize that a "normal life" is made up of much more than food.

Self-Pity

Another normal-but-unpleasant emotion you may experience is self-pity. Here you have a child who has been sick, who has a disease he will never outgrow, and you're feeling sorry for yourself. Don't feel guilty about that!

Nearly every parent feels some self-pity shortly after the diagnosis. And why not? All the other parents get to whip up a quick box of macaroni-and-cheese for dinner, drive through a fast-food restaurant without making several calls before-hand, and shove a bunch of crackers in the kid's fist when he's whining in the car. *Their* biggest dietary concern is making sure their kids' pizza has enough pep-peroni on it to count as a source of protein. So go ahead . . . feel a little sorry for yourself, because it *is* tough. But then get over it and move on, because your family needs you. Besides, you have some work to do to prepare yourself—and your child—for a happy, healthy gluten-free life.

Guilt

Many parents are guilt-ridden, and will ask, "What did I do to give my child this condition?" Beyond the basic physiology of the birds and the bees, the answer is *nothing*. Certainly you did nothing *wrong*. Celiac disease is a genetic condition, so there *is* a biological connection, and someone *did* pass a gene along to the child. But there is certainly no reason to wallow in guilt, because nothing could have been done differently to avoid the condition.

Acceptance

Yes, you will learn to accept the diagnosis, and you will one day look back and wonder why it seemed so overwhelming at first. While some of the other emotions may rear their ugly heads again from time to time, you will realize that it's a lot more fun to focus on your child's activities, school projects, friends, sports, accomplishments, and virtues than it is to spend your energy worrying about his diagnosis.

Am I Doing Something Wrong?
It Seems Too Easy . . .

Ah, this is when you know you've finally made it.

There comes a time when parents who have become accustomed to dealing with their child's gluten-free diet wonder if they're doing something wrong because it seems too easy. Those feelings of self-doubt are usually triggered by a conversation with a parent who is still in the panic phase—still trying to figure out what, besides Fritos, they can feed their child, and how their lives will ever return to "normal." The experienced parent will think, "Gee, I really don't give any thought to it anymore. I wonder if I'm being too lax, or if I'm missing something here. It's just really not that tough."

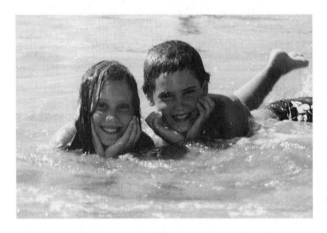

When this happens to you, don't question yourself. Just enjoy the peace of mind, and realize you have acclimated to your new lifestyle. With the realization that you have that monkey off your back, you may want to take some time to help someone else with a difficult situation, and revel in the satisfaction that will bring.

4

The First Few Steps

Once you have gotten over the initial shock of your child's diagnosis, the first step is to educate yourself and the people around you. Yes, it seems overwhelming at first, but the less you understand about celiac disease, the scarier it is.

Do Your Homework

Take a few weeks to peruse the Internet for information on celiac disease. There are several good websites with current research, product information, and resources. At the end of this book you'll also find a Resource Guide that will refer you to several good sources of online and print information, as well as a list of helpful publications.

Get Organized

There is *a lot* of information to digest, and you will be well served to stay organized. Start a binder or file with sections for information on:
- gluten-free foods,
- manufacturers' contact information and correspondence,
- correspondence with restaurants,

"We're just getting started with the gluten-free diet. We're looking for ANY tips that will make it easier"
—Dan and Debbie F.

- resources (mail order food companies, for instance),
- and organizations.

See Chapter 11 for more information on collecting and organizing information.

Contact Support Groups

Get in touch with celiac disease organizations such as Celiac Disease Foundation, Celiac Sprue Association, and Gluten Intolerance Group. (See the Resource Guide for contact information.) They will send you important information that will help you get started with the diet. They also have local support groups that hold regular meetings that you may wish to attend. Some parents find these meetings valuable because they find that their child is not alone in their condition; many enjoy the meetings because they feature knowledgeable speakers; others take pleasure in the camaraderie that can result from attending the meetings.

The Internet also offers opportunities for joining support groups and sharing information. In addition to websites that offer a myriad of information and services, there is a celiac LISTSERV (see Resource Guide), which offers opportunities for members to share information, ask questions, and voice opinions. Remember, though, that not *all* of the people submitting information to the LISTSERV—or to websites, for that matter—are experts. Some of the information must be taken with a grain (gluten-free, of course) of salt.

Don't Be Afraid to Feed Your Kid

True, the list of foods your child has to avoid for life is very long. But there is a much longer list of foods that your child *can* eat without a problem.

First, check out the lists of safe and forbidden foods in Chapter 11 (pages 62-66), and head to the grocery store to stock up on products that your child likes. Also, try out some of the gluten-free staples such as bread, pasta, and mixes for baked goods that are available from specialty stores and by phone or Internet order. (See the Resource Guide for addresses.) Then turn to the "Quick Meal Ideas" in Chapter 12 (pages 72-78). Here you will find more than enough tasty options for meals and snacks to keep your child happily fed until you feel knowledgeable enough to confidently plan your own menus again.

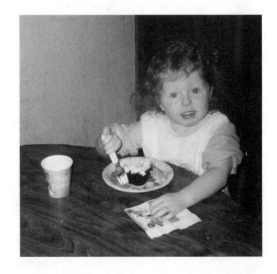

5 Attitude is Life . . .

Deal with It;
Don't Dwell on It

"Annie was just diagnosed last week, and I find myself coddling her, trying to make up for the diagnosis in some way. I'm still reeling with emotion, and I feel overwhelmed. Will it ever get easier?"
—Darryl S.

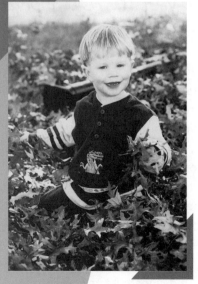

Keep It In Perspective

Deal with it; don't dwell on it: That's our mantra throughout this book. We have seen many parents over the years get so caught up with the "inconveniences" of having a child with celiac disease that it becomes a negative, controlling force in their lives. Yes, it's difficult at first, and it *is* a family affair, affecting everyone in the family greatly. But how you deal with it is going to influence your child's emotions and behavior, and can have long-lasting effects. Remember, your child's diet is a small part of his life; it shouldn't be the entire focus.

Shortly after diagnosis, your child is experiencing many physical and emotional changes. Chances are, he was very sick, and you were doting over him, genuinely concerned about whether he was even going to live through the ordeal. That has probably created some interesting dynamics: you had a *very* sick child, and in some cases, it was grave; it will be difficult for you to let go of that fear and concern at first.

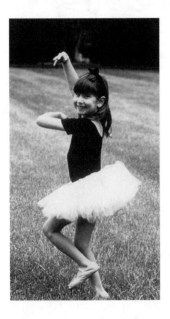

As for your child, he has been getting a lot of attention from parents and doctors, and may have mixed emotions about getting better!

Fortunately, you should see fairly quick improvement in his physical health once you start a gluten-free diet. And although most physicians agree that there are behavioral issues when a celiac child is still on a gluten-containing diet, many of these, if not all, will disappear quickly after beginning a gluten-free diet.

There will, however, be periods of frustration and irritability, and the temptation to let him have a birthday cupcake or holiday cookie. Hang in there, and whatever you do, don't let him cheat! Not only will it cause physical harm, but it is sending him a signal that you are going to be inconsistent about enforcing his diet. You all need to take this diet very seriously, and you must commit yourselves to being 100 percent gluten-free. Be supportive during these periods of frustration; let him know his feelings are completely normal. But urge him, especially by example, to move forward, discovering the wonderful new world of gluten-free living.

Be Optimistic, Even If You Have to Fake It at First

Have you ever pretended to feel a certain way, for whatever reason, and found that eventually you *actually feel* that way? It's a wonderful power that our brains have, and most of us are not even aware of it. Of course, it can be used for positive feelings or negative ones, but for the purpose of this book, we'll focus on "pretending" to be optimistic.

Try thinking of the diagnosis and your child's condition as a challenge. Don't let it knock you down (at least not for long). Come up with reasons to think of this as a good thing—maybe it's bringing you and your child, or you and your spouse, closer together. Maybe it's causing you to focus on a healthier diet. Perhaps it's forcing you to focus less on work and more on your family. If you need to, write down the reasons that this could be a good thing in your life. Memorize them. Believe them. You will be amazed at how your behavior and sincere feelings will follow.

The truth is that the diagnosis of celiac disease in our children is far harder on us parents than it is on our children. We tend to think of the things *we* ate as children. We tend to focus on what they're *missing*. But you know what? They don't *know* what they're missing! You could be feeding them daffodils every day, and they wouldn't know what they were missing out on. Sure, at first they know, especially if they're older. But after they adjust to their lifestyle, it's nothing more than a "cultural" difference. Vegetarians don't eat meat. They don't focus on the steak and pork chops they're missing; they take pleasure in the wonderful assortment of foods that they do enjoy.

It's our disappointment for our children that makes this so difficult—so learn to see the positive, and it will be reflected in your child's optimistic views and behaviors. Remember that a positive attitude for life begins in their earliest years.

They Are Different, and That's Okay!

When parents of newly diagnosed kids call, one of the first things they always say is, "I'm so worried he'll grow up feeling *different* from the other kids."

It's a natural response. As adults, we have all felt "different" at one time or another, and that feeling has made us feel uncomfortable. We make the assumption that feeling "different" is painful. As parents, we want to spare our children the heartache that we *anticipate* they'll feel.

> *"I'm afraid people will treat Jenna differently because her diet may seem strange to them. I don't want her to feel abnormal. What can I do to make it so she doesn't feel so different?"*
> —Mike J.

The fact is, they *are* different—but no different from someone with an allergy to chocolate or peanuts. No different from the child whose recess activities are limited due to asthma. No different from the child with a different religious or ethnic background.

Our children need to know that they *are* different, and that's okay. If you lead them to believe they're *no* different from anyone else, they're surely going to wonder why *everyone else* eats such peculiar stuff. It will skew their entire sense of reality, because the reality is that *they* are the ones with the "different" diet. They need to learn to deal with that. It's not a bad thing, nor is it anything to shield them from.

Don't Keep Him in a Bubble

It's natural to want to protect your child, and it may take some time to feel comfortable enough with the diet to venture out. It may seem at first that you need to forego dinner at friends' houses or restaurants. You may think you should eliminate travel from your activities, keep your child home while the other kids go away to camp, or tell him he can't go to a pizza party.

Don't do that to yourself or to your kids. Yes, every time you venture outside the safety of your gluten-friendly kitchen, you're taking a risk that he will get some gluten. And yes, it's important to be as diligent as you can about ensuring a 100 percent gluten-free diet. So how do you resolve that paradox? You could keep your child in a bubble—but it seems to me that it's worse to grow up in isolation than to take the risk that he may get a small bit of gluten. It's important to remember an almost universal goal of raising children: to teach our kids to live successfully in the world. To learn about their world, they have to be immersed in it.

> *"It seems like it would just be easier to keep Danny at home. I could home-school him, and then I wouldn't have to worry. I really don't know how we're ever going to get out of this house again!"*
> —Tammy L.

Teach Your Child to Have a Positive Attitude

Attitudes are contagious. So the first and most important thing is to remember that your child is *always* watching how you handle situations—and you can bet he'll be tuning in to how you deal with his condition.

Tell your child that *he is in control of how he feels.* He can choose to feel sad, or he can choose to feel happy. Of course, we all feel sad sometimes, sadness is perfectly justified when you're first finding out you have celiac disease. It's important that your child understands that, and isn't *too* quick to shrug off or bury negative emotions. Some of the most important lessons children learn involve managing emotions, especially "unpleasant" ones.

Your child may feel sad when he can't eat something the other kids are eating, or when a friend or relative "just doesn't get it." Sympathize,

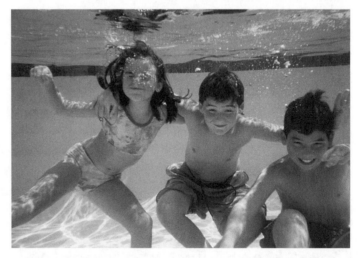

but don't let him dwell on it. Teach him that he can *choose* to pull himself out of that gloomy feeling by thinking of how lucky he is to be able to eat chocolate or other yummy things that some people can't eat. Help him to focus on the positive things—not only concerning celiac disease, but other positive attributes that he has, or exciting things going on in his life.

Don't Make a Big Deal of It to Him

Other than discussing food choices and other practical matters associated with celiac disease, try not to make this a huge issue in your life. Of course it *is*, but for your child's sake, pretend it isn't. Sometimes it's tough not to make a big deal of it, because you assume that it will have the same impact on your child's life as it has on yours. It doesn't. For the most part, sports or activities, school, and friends are what kids want to think about—and what they *should* be thinking about.

A couple of times, in an attempt to be sensitive and communicative, we have tried asking Tyler how it makes him feel to have celiac disease. We expected to hear how emotionally devastating it is, how angry he is at that unknown descendant who passed him the "inferior" gene. Instead, he looked at us as though we had the I.Q. of an oyster, and said, "It doesn't feel like anything. It's no big deal."

Don't Let Him Feel Like a Burden — Obvious? Not Always

"Don't let your child feel like a burden" sounds like elementary psychology, and appears to be blatantly obvious. But picture yourself at the end of a long week, tired from a busy day, ready to relax, and you hear, "Mommy, I don't have any bread left. Can we make some?" Surely you'll be tempted to roll your eyes and give a heavy sigh—a perfectly natural reaction. This is where you'll be cursing all of your friends who can just make a quick trip to the grocery store. Go ahead and curse them, but do it to yourself.

The last thing you want is for your child to think that he is causing you extra stress because of his diet. Kids are so perceptive! You don't have to say anything. They'll read it in your eyes, or your body language, especially if they're looking for it because they've suspected in the past that their diet creates a burden. Muster any energy you have left, give him a big smile, and pull out the trusty bread maker. (Or offer a yummy alternative.)

Celiac Disease Is Not a Four-Letter Word

Although celiac disease is not a four-letter word, people sure do *act* like it is! What is it about this condition that makes people squirm? Relatives can have every classic symptom, yet they refuse to be tested. It can't be that the condition involves the "insides," and is therefore too private in nature. After all, people are

"Christopher had chronic diarrhea, and because celiac disease runs in our family, we suggested to our pediatrician that he should do an antibody screening. But he said that because Christopher was normal height and weight, there was no reason to test him. Why won't he just do the test?"
—Lynnette C.

• • •

"Some people would rather hear that they have to take a pill every day of their lives, than to hear that they have to change their diet!"
—Elaine Monarch,
Celiac Disease Foundation

happy to discuss their Crohn's disease, ulcerative colitis, hair loss, prostate problems, and infertility. No, it's something much less tangible, and much more subtle.

Even many doctors are hesitant to accept celiac disease. I have seen several cases in which celiac disease runs in the family, and a child has classic symptoms; parents ask for their child to be tested, and the doctor refuses. WHY? The blood test is not expensive, it's noninvasive, and it's an excellent initial screening. But there's something about celiac disease that people want to avoid.

Be aware of this fact, but don't buy into it. There is nothing to be ashamed of, and nothing to be embarrassed about. While there is no need to wear a badge of celiac disease, be aware of how your child may be picking up on the stigma, and be careful that your child never feels as though his condition is something to hide.

Realize You Have New Commitments

Your new gluten-free lifestyle will require you to spend more time preparing, planning, cooking, educating, and volunteering your time.

The best way to help your child ease into a gluten-free lifestyle is for you to volunteer as often as you can to help with, if not lead, school-related and extracurricular activities. If you can, chaperone field trips and camping expeditions, volunteer to help with lunch time at school (only if your school has volunteers; you don't want to be the one parent there—it may make your child feel even more "different"). Divide this extra effort between husband and wife, if possible. Dads are just as good (or better) at chaperoning on field trips as moms are! It's your job to do everything in your power to keep your child happy and healthy. When you have a child with celiac disease, that may mean putting in a little extra effort at times.

6

*S*hould the Entire Family be Gluten-Free?

"I don't want David to see the rest of the family eating things that he can't eat, so I'm thinking about getting rid of everything in the house that has gluten in it, and making the entire house gluten-free. Would that make it easier for him to deal with the diet?"
—Cindy P.

Nearly every family that has a member who has celiac disease considers turning the entire house into a gluten-free zone. Is it necessary to do so? Is it "easier" on everyone? Well, it is definitely not *necessary* for the entire family to be gluten-free. There are, in fact, pros and cons to both sides.

The Pros

The pros of having an entirely gluten-free family are that it's simpler at menu-planning time, shopping is less cumbersome, it's easier to keep a gluten-free kitchen, there is little or no possibility of accidental contamination or ingestion, and there's no temptation for your child to cheat (at home). You also avoid the resentment that your celiac child may feel when the rest of the family is eating something that she can't eat.

The Cons

Remember, in solving one problem, you can create another. If the entire family goes gluten-free, your non-celiac kids (and spouse!) may begin to resent the celiac child for imposing the diet on the family.

Perhaps the most important argument against having the entire family lead a completely gluten-free lifestyle is that *it simply isn't reality*. Kids with celiac disease have to learn to live in a gluten-laden world, and what safer, more controlled place to learn than in the home? Yes, menu-planning is more difficult when you have to cook "both ways," and yes, the child on the gluten-free diet is likely to feel pangs of jealousy and even isolation. But there are ways to soften those blows, yet still live in a "real" world surrounded by gluten.

Finding a Happy Medium

Perhaps the best compromise is to have the family be *relatively* gluten-free. Try to eat the same types of meals, with a small portion being different when necessary. For instance, if it's spaghetti night, you might want to make gluten-free pasta for everyone. But if not, it's okay to have everyone eat gluten-containing spaghetti with the one child eating gluten-free pasta (be sure to use separate pots, colanders, and serving utensils). The entire family can use the same gluten-free spaghetti sauce and parmesan, and people will hardly notice that one child is eating a different type of pasta. Just make sure that your child's meal and the family's meal are pretty much the same. You don't want to be eating lasagna and offering her lima beans.

Try to find gluten-free staple items that everyone likes—yogurt, salad dressings, condiments, sauces, and other frequently used foods and accouterments. That way the possibility of cross-contamination or accidental gluten ingestion is minimized, your celiac child doesn't feel ostracized, and you won't need to convert the spare bedroom into a pantry to accommodate two sets of every type of food.

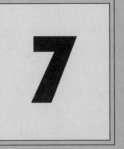

7

Talking to Your Children about Celiac Disease

"Tiffany was diagnosed a month ago. She's only three years old, and I figured she was too young to understand, so I've just been taking charge of her diet and I haven't talked to her about celiac disease. I thought maybe I'd wait until she's four. My husband thinks we should do it now. What's the right age?"
—Lynn and John T.

Educating Your Child

Whether your child is two or twelve, you need to start talking to him about his diet *now*. Don't use made-up words, and don't be afraid to use big words. Understanding is a tool that benefits both children and adults, although the extent of information provided will vary with the age of your child. It's important to *give your child both an understanding and control of his diet so the diet doesn't control him!*

Regardless of his age, your child is obviously aware that he has been sick, gone through testing, his parents have been concerned, and that doctors have been doing all sorts of crazy things to him. Once the diagnosis is established, it's time to explain to him that all of that is behind him now, and that he's going to start feeling a lot better, starting right away!

Open the conversation by explaining that he has a condition called celiac disease. How extensive this conversation will be depends upon the age of your child, of course, but give him as much information as he seems to want. Don't pout, cry, or look sad or apologetic when you talk about it! Explain that some people can't eat sugar, others can't eat chocolate, and he can't eat gluten. Surely you know someone who has a dietary restriction that you can point out as an example. Keep remembering, and expressing to him, that the *good* thing is he's going to start feeling better right away!

When you first start talking about gluten, make sure you have a quick "sound bite" to describe it. For instance, you might say, "You can't eat gluten. Gluten is in wheat, oats, rye, and barley." (You might want to add "malt" to the list, too. Malt is made from barley, but how many kids *or* adults know that?) Every time you refer to "gluten," try to follow it up with the identical phrase: "gluten is in wheat, oats, rye, and barley (malt)." Repeat the phrase every time the key word (gluten) is mentioned, and, even if your child doesn't have a clue what these things are, he'll learn the words. This is useful so that he will be able to repeat them to others as necessary. It's important that he can say the words, even if he doesn't understand what they mean.

It is through actions such as telling others about the disease that your child will begin managing his own condition. Of course it is also important to talk with your child about what items *contain* gluten, such

If Your Child Has a Disability

If your child has difficulty communicating due to Down syndrome, autism, or another disability, consider providing him with a card that explains that

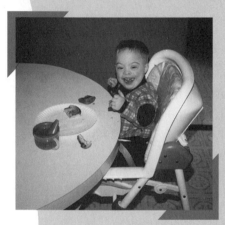

he can't eat wheat, oats, rye, and barley (malt). Over time, teach him to show it to people who may offer him food. For example, when your child goes to a friend's house, have him offer the card to the parent in charge. In the beginning, you may need to use hand-over-hand guidance to prompt him to show the card at appropriate times. As time goes on, you might prompt him with the word "card" or wait to see whether he will remember to show the card on his own. The goal is for him to eventually be independent in recognizing people who need to know about the foods he cannot eat.

If your child uses an alternative or augmentative communication system, include information about your child's food restrictions in his communication system. That way, he can just hit the button on his communication device to explain what he can or can't eat, or turn to the appropriate page in his communication book.

as cookies, bread, and cereal. But getting him to think and talk in "sound bites" (or offer an explanatory card) will help him communicate his condition and restrictions to others, even before he fully understands the complexities of the diet.

How You Might Bring It Up with Your Young Child

It's a lot easier to explain celiac disease to older children than to younger ones (although older kids pose additional challenges in terms of cheating), so we have outlined an example of how you might begin to explain celiac disease and gluten to younger kids. Remember, keep that positive attitude!

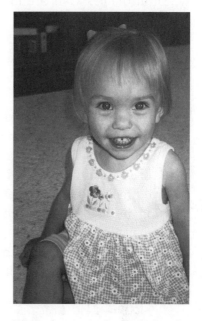

Ages One to Six:

"Honey, you know we've been going to see Dr. B. a whole bunch lately, right? Well, he is *so* smart that he figured out what we can do to make you feel better!" (Keep that smile and enthusiasm!) "See, you have this thing called celiac disease. That's why you weren't feeling good, but now that we know what it is, you're going to start feeling much better! Celiac disease just means there are some things you can't eat, but there are *lots* of things you *can* eat! Let's go in the pantry right now and find some gluten-free snacks together."

At this point, let him point out something he wants. Chances are, he'll pick something with gluten. Now's your chance to say, "Oh, that looks really yummy. But that has gluten in it—gluten is in wheat, oats, rye, and barley (malt). Let's see what we have that doesn't have gluten in it. . . ." (This is when you pick up a gluten-free candy bar or something *really* yummy that you've stashed for this very moment.)

Of course, your discussions will evolve, and there is a steep learning curve for everyone involved. Many of the implications of having a dietary restriction do not become immediately clear. Many such issues will emerge gradually over time and will require learning and adaptation for some time to come. For instance, you just learned something new from the monologue above, Rule Number One: always have an alternative (and better tasting) snack handy. But we'll talk more about that in later chapters.

'amiliar Examples

ᴇ trying to explain to your child that gluten is in wheat, oats, (malt), remember that he probably doesn't know exactly what ᴌean. One technique to help him understand the meaning of the ᵥ. ᴧk each grain with a product he knows. For instance, "Wheat is in the brea. ᴇ used to eat. It's also in crackers, spaghetti, cakes, and cookies. But now we'll be making special cookies (bread, spaghetti, etc.) that don't have any wheat in them." "Oats are in oatmeal," and so on.

Activities for Young Kids

Activities are an effective learning tool for young children, and a great way for young kids to become involved in the process of learning about the gluten-free diet. It's a good idea to involve all of your children in the activities, even those who are not on a gluten-free diet. Not only will they learn about the diet too, but it will help all the family members feel that "we're all in this together."

There are activity books available that are geared toward the gluten-free child, or you can come up with your own. One suggestion is to have your child help you make a food booklet or flashcards with "good" foods and "bad" foods. Cooking magazines and old cookbooks are loaded with colorful pictures. You can paste the pictures onto colored paper or colorful cloth scraps, and bind them together with yarn or rings that snap closed. You can even use the booklet as a resource for friends and family!

"Just the Facts, Ma'am" Approach for Older Kids

How you talk with your older child depends upon the relationship you have and the responses you get throughout the conversation. Basically, though, older kids would prefer you just cut to the chase.

Your child is going to want the basic facts. Elaborate as you'd like, but remember to include the following basic elements:

- You have celiac disease.
- This is what celiac disease is.
- That's why you haven't felt well.
- Kids with celiac disease can't eat gluten.
- Gluten is in wheat, oats, rye, and barley (malt).
- Here are some lists of things that are okay to eat, and things that are not.
- If you get even a tiny bit of gluten, it does really bad things to you internally.
- You need to learn how to say, "No thank you."
- If you don't know for sure, don't eat it.
- It may not be easy, but we'll help you through it.

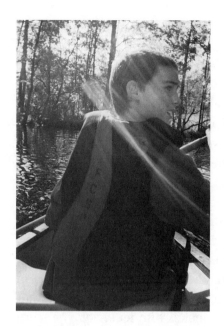

Your discussions with older kids are important, but it's even more important to help them research the condition on their own. The more they know, the less scary it will be, and learning about it is the first step in taking responsibility for their own health. For many older children, anything their parents tell them is subject to question until verified by another source. There are a number of good websites and various written materials listed in the back of this book that can help.

It is important for you to understand that, shortly after being diagnosed, older children may go through many of the same emotions that parents experience (described in Chapter Three). If you're aware of these normal-but-not-always-pleasant emotions, you will likely be more patient and supportive during your interactions with your child.

"If You Feel Bad, You Must Have Gotten Gluten"

Talking with your child about celiac disease is an ongoing process—something you discuss in different ways as his level of understanding (and yours) grows. I do *not* want to give the impression that you should dwell on the subject, nor should you make a huge deal out of it (in fact, I believe quite the opposite). But there are some things you want to "condition in," so to speak.

For instance, especially in the beginning, when you refer to gluten, you need to remind your child that he can't eat gluten. You might want to say something like, "Remember, you can't eat gluten. It makes you feel icky." (Okay, if he's thirteen, you may want to choose a word other than "icky.") You may feel like you're being redundant, repetitive, and even a nag. And you *are!* But think about how many dozens of times you've said, "Don't run with a sucker in your mouth," and yet 99 percent of the time when your kids put a sucker in their mouth, it's as though their transmission automatically kicks into "RUN" mode. Some things are so important that they just have to be repeated. It may not be that your children forgot, or even that they're intentionally defying or ignoring you—it's that their knowledge of that association hasn't gone to a deep, subliminal level yet.

It may be helpful to think about how associations between events are developed. Some associations are conditioned in very early. For instance, cry = attention from a parent. Mommy talking on phone = ask for something and chances are good that you'll get it. These aren't associations that children are consciously aware of. Rather, these associations develop through observation. In other words, they are conditioned by experience. Children observe that, sure enough, when Mommy has that thing on her ear and is deep in conversation, she tends to nod when interrupted and asked a question. The same type of process is necessary for conditioning children that "gluten makes them feel icky." You want this lesson to be so ingrained in their head that they come to believe it, deep down inside, at

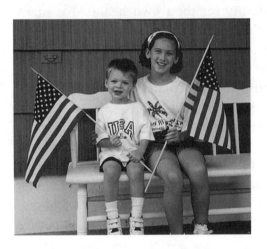

the level where their subconscious is also supposed to be chanting, "hit brother = time-out."

The key words in the last sentence were, "come to believe it." If your child is younger than a teen, you still have some influence over what he believes. This is where conditioning comes in again. I believe there is great power in conditioning your child to believe that gluten makes him feel icky. The truth is, eating gluten is not *always* going to make him feel icky, and this can cre-

ate some difficulties when you're trying to convince him how awful gluten is for his body. So, in an effort to maximize your child's understanding of this unpleasant reality, you may want to take advantage of any time he *does* feel icky, and blame it on gluten. With this necessary goal in mind, it doesn't really matter if it's the flu, a "regular ol' tummy ache," food poisoning, or a mild headache. When he complains of symptoms, reply with, "Oh, honey, I am so sorry to hear you don't feel well. Maybe you accidentally got some gluten. It makes you feel icky, you know." As the association becomes clearer, the likelihood that he will try to sneak some gluten in the future is diminished.

Read Labels Together — Even If He Can't Read Yet

Whether your child can read or not, it is important to read the product labels together. I know that sounds silly. If he can't read, why would you have him read a label with you? The answer is dual purpose. Reading labels with your child not only involves him in the decision-making process, it also helps him get in the habit of looking at labels on packages. That conditioning thing again.

Of course, you don't ask him to read the words aloud to you, but you can hold the package together, point to each word on the ingredients list, and when you get to, for instance, "wheat," you say, "wheat—nope. Can't eat wheat, because wheat has gluten in it." You may even want to finish with, "Gluten makes you feel icky." Your continual and repetitive statements of these basic concepts really will help increase your child's understanding of, and belief in, the impact of gluten on his body. Repetition is a fundamental aspect of the conditioning process.

How to Say "No Thank You"

Unfortunately, there *will* be the well-meaning grandparent or auntie who slips your child a cookie and says with a conspiratorial wink, "Don't tell Mommy and Daddy." There will also be people who are completely unaware of your child's condition, and, with the best of intentions, will offer him something he can't eat. At holidays, it seems as if people come swarming from nowhere to offer children candy canes or other treats that may or may not be safe.

It is very important to talk with your child about temptation and why people will tempt him. Explain that Grandma means well, but that she just doesn't understand how bad gluten is for him. Tell him that the elves offering cookies just don't know that he can't eat those things. But remind him of how very important it is not to eat things that might have gluten in them.

Teach him to say, "No thank you" without apology, explanation, or embarrassment. There are times when saying anything further can be awkward and it certainly isn't necessary. Of course if he *wants* to explain, that's fine. But stress that it's okay just to politely refuse the treat. And if you're there, be sure to offer a tasty alternative.

Let Him Know There Are Alternatives: Do the "Treat Trade"

When discussing your child's dietary restrictions, make sure he knows that there are always tasty alternatives. Be sure to reinforce this with your actions. You may have to get creative sometimes, and short notice can be a real curse— but it's important to always offer some sort of an alternative when your child is in a situation in which he can't eat something. For instance, if the other kids are eating birthday cupcakes and you didn't have time to make gluten-free cupcakes, offer him a candy bar. If the other kids are eating Christmas cookies, make sure he has his favorite treat available. When you see the disappointment on his face because all the

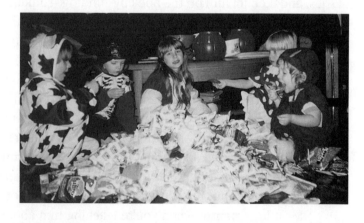

other kids get to have pizza, make him his favorite meal—preferably his gluten-free pizza. This technique is most effective if the alternative is similar to what the other kids are eating.

It can also help if the alternative is just a little bit "better" than what the other kids get. When the other kids in Tyler's class were eating birthday cake and he got a Snicker's Bar, they all complained that he always got the "good" stuff!

How the food looks is just as important as how it tastes. If the other kids are having a pizza party and you send your child with his own pizza, it better look "right." If not, you can be sure he will hide it, toss it, and come home famished and embarrassed.

Okay, It's Time to Eat!

So you've had your little heart-to-heart, and your child is saying, "Yeah, yeah, whatever. Celiac schmeliac. Let's EAT!" Start by asking him to choose a food he'd like to eat. After he chooses something, ask him if he thinks it has gluten in it. Remind him that gluten is in wheat, oats, rye, and barley (malt). Yes, of course

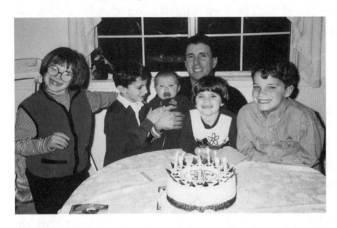

I know that he doesn't know what these things are! That's not the point! The point is that in asking him this question you are encouraging him to think about what he can and can't eat.

Let him choose a few items, and if they contain gluten, point out why they're not okay to eat: "No, those cookies have flour in them. That means they have gluten." Give him a couple of tries, and then let him off the hook by "finding" something you've hidden away—the yummiest gluten-free treat you can think of! In the beginning, this activity should be at least a daily exercise, if not something you do every time he wants a snack. Repetition and familiarity are keys to getting started with this new lifestyle.

While the diagnosis is still fresh, he may be wondering if he's ever going to get a "normal" meal! It's important to explain that dinners *will* be a little different now, and be sure to involve him in the menu-planning process. This will be tough at first, at least until you've figured out how to prepare gluten-free pasta, pizza, and other highly requested menu items. But it is very important to his adaptation to at least let him *think* he's helping plan the menus, especially if there are things he happens to like that are gluten-free, such as salad or rice.

Most importantly, when you're teaching him about eating gluten-free, don't ever let him think that this dietary lifestyle is optional. Remind him that gluten will make him feel icky, and teach him the safest decision tool, "If you don't know, don't eat it."

Talking to the Other Kids in the Family

If there are siblings, it's important to talk with them about celiac disease and the new diet for the child with celiac disease. Depending upon the siblings' age(s) and relationships, they may have all sorts of questions, fears, and other feelings that need to be discussed. A diagnosis of one child in a family has an emotional impact on all family members. Be aware that your nondiagnosed children could be feeling any of the following emotions:

> *"I know I need to talk to Renee's little brother about Renee's condition, but I'm afraid it might scare him. Will he be afraid she's going to die? Will he be afraid he had it too? How do we talk to the other kids in the family about this?"*
> —Rebecca B.

- Fear:
    - Am I going to get it?
    - Can I catch it?
    - Is my brother/sister going to die?
- Resentment:
    - He gets "special" attention and I don't.
    - He gets better treats than I do (especially common when you're making a treat-trade and the child with celiac disease gets a really yummy treat).
    - Parents care more about him than me because he's different.
- Sadness or pity:
    - He has a special diet and can't eat all of the really good stuff that many people can.

And then again, because siblings will be siblings, they may be tempted to make fun of him, tease him, or wave a greasy doughnut under his nose.

It's important for siblings to understand which foods are safe, which are not, and how important it is to take the diet seriously. Include them in all of your family discussions about celiac disease, so that they too can make wise food choices for your child.

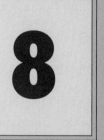

8

Give Your Child Control of Her Diet!

It's Your Responsibility to Give Your Child the Responsibility

It's funny. We teach our kids to dress themselves, to brush their own teeth, to go to the potty by themselves. . . . But when it comes to choosing what they eat, no sirree, Mommy will do that for you, thank you very much. Especially when the food they eat can make them very sick.

Yet, just as it's our job as parents to teach our children not to run out into the street, it's our responsibility to teach *them* to take responsibility for their diet. Remember, our job as parents, as difficult as it is for some of us to accept, is to raise our children in a loving, protective environment so that they can (ugh) *leave* us someday! Our instincts tell us to protect them, to control their environment so that nothing will hurt them. That's not too hard at three, but at thirteen, the very word "control" will drive a stake right through the heart of your relationship with your child.

It is important that children learn to size up risks and avoid or ignore them. They need to know that you trust them to take care of themselves—and you need to trust them to do so. However, getting to that point is a process that will take time for both sides.

As our children grow, they need to be able to:

- Identify, assess, and handle temptations and risks;
- Handle peer pressure;
- Handle social situations in which gluten is present;
- Prepare in advance for social functions in which there may be no gluten-free alternatives;
- Select foods in social settings and at the grocery store;
- Plan healthy, well-balanced gluten-free meals;
- Cook;
- Understand the consequences of cheating or accidental ingestion;
- Educate the people around them about celiac disease and the gluten-free diet.

It's Never Too Early

Whether your child is a toddler or a teen, let her know that she is responsible for her diet. *If she doesn't feel in control of her diet, her diet will control her.*

Helping your child to take control of her diet is crucial to her physical and emotional well-being, so you might as well start as soon as possible. Don't think

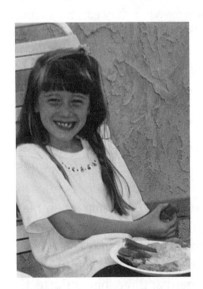

you're doing her any favors by making all of her decisions for her, even if she is very young. In fact, you're taking away her sense of control, not to mention the fact that she's not learning to feed herself. Remember the wise Native American saying: "If you give a person a fish, he will eat for a day. If you teach a person to fish, he will eat for a lifetime."

The earlier you give your child responsibility for her diet, the better off she'll be. It will also be easier for you in the long run. You will relax knowing that she understands the gluten-free diet and can make responsible, healthy choices. More importantly, being responsible for her own diet will give your child confidence; she will know that she is capable of determining whether or not a food is gluten-free. In addition, at a subconscious level, she will have taken control of her condition, rather than letting it control her.

Things Children Can Do Right Away to Take Control

Menu Planning

Sometimes kids can be picky eaters. Toss into the equation the fact that your child's diet is severely limited, and meal planning can be frustrating, to say the least. Get your child involved in the meal-planning process! Not only will you be teaching her about the foods she can and can't eat, but you'll be working *together* to come up with a menu that pleases everyone. (The rule at our house is if you plan it, you eat it. No designating Tuesday as "fish night," and then deciding you don't like fish that week.) See Chapter 12 (pg. 72) for menu suggestions.

Cooking

Kids are never too young to start helping in the kitchen. Of course, it's usually a lot easier and cleaner if they *don't* help, but it's important that children learn to prepare their own foods. Get all of the kids involved. A big part of the learning process, especially if you have other kids who are not gluten-free, is learning how to avoid contaminating utensils and cooking surfaces (see Chapter 10). By the time your child is eight, there will be many meals she can make on her own. The benefits are many: it makes it easier on you, it's fun for your children, and you're teaching them to be independent. Remember, cleaning up the kitchen after you cook is one of the most important rules!

Packing Lunches

Have your child pack her own lunch, at least every now and then. You may want to check to make sure she doesn't go off to school with a solid meal of chips, candy bars, and "fruit" juice—but having her pack her own lunch will help you out and reinforce what she's learning about making good food choices. We offer gluten-free suggestions for lunches and other meals in Chapter 12.

Calling Manufacturers

Calling manufacturers to ask whether their products contain gluten is going to be something you and your child do frequently, so you might as well start involving your child at an early age. Fortunately, many large food manufacturers and distributors now have lists of gluten-free products, and can tell you over the phone whether or not their products are gluten-free. (A far cry from just a few years ago when even the most knowledgeable customer service reps would confidently inform me, "Oh yes, honey, you may not know this, but gluten is another word for sugar. Most of our products *do* contain sugar and should be avoided by diabetics.")

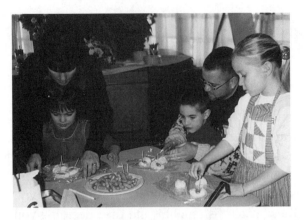

Every now and then you'll get someone who hasn't heard of gluten, and you'll need to work your way to their nutritionist or dietitian. But for the most part, customer service reps who answer the phone can tell you whether or not their products contain gluten.

To help your child get the hang of this process, make sure her first few calls are to companies whose customer service reps have a gluten-free list in front of them. You'll want to "scout" out those companies in advance. (Don't tell your child you've already called the company, because she'll feel you don't trust her. You'll deflate her sense of purpose.) But when you've found a company with knowledgeable customer service reps at the other end, suggest to your child that she call about a product, and let her take it from there. Remind her to take notes and keep the information in your personalized product listing that you keep at home (suggested in Chapter 11).

Condition Your Child to Avoid Gluten

This entire chapter dealt with giving your child responsibility for her diet. But let go completely? No way! No matter how much "discussing," how much preaching, or how much begging you do, there's the possibility— read that as "likelihood"—that your child won't initially truly fathom the importance of always selecting safe, gluten-free foods. This almost always occurs in people with any type of dietary restriction.

Thanks to the wonders of the human body, you still have some tricks up your sleeve to help drive the point home. People with celiac disease have a simple built-in negative reinforcement clause—when they eat gluten, they feel bad.

Use this to your advantage! As I've mentioned earlier, we tricked our son when he was very young in an effort to condition him to avoid gluten. And it worked! Every time he hurt—whether it was a tummy ache, stubbed toe, or a headache, we said, "Uh oh, you must have gotten some gluten. We'll have to be more careful next time." In effect, we conditioned him to avoid gluten by teaching him that it caused discomfort. And for what it's worth, if the proof is in the gluten-free pudding, today we couldn't pay him to eat gluten.

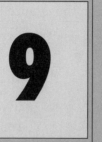

Dealing with Family and Friends

You think it was tough talking to your kid about celiac disease? Ha! Kids are quick studies compared to many adult relatives, friends, teachers, and other people you encounter.

Educating the adults in your life is, perhaps, one of the most difficult aspects of having a child with celiac disease. Because there is so little awareness of celiac disease, responses from family and friends range from confusion (you'll recognize this response because as you're explaining it, their eyes glaze over and they say, "huh" a lot), to complete understanding (sorry, this is rare) to histrionic horror (usually exhibited by grandmothers who, at the word "disease," break down and sob), to disbelief (particularly common if you're known to exaggerate from time to time).

Educate Your Family and Friends

You do not need to make an announcement when you walk into a room and declare to everyone that your child is on a special diet. I say this facetiously, yet we know many parents of celiac kids who do just that! They feel that they're doing "the right thing" by letting everyone know about the dietary restriction, thereby reducing the chance that someone

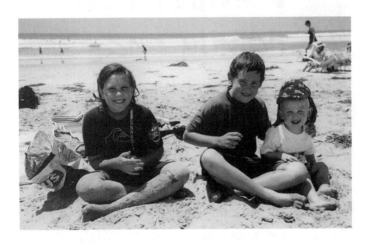

will slip their child a cookie. But keep in mind that your child is listening, and no matter how young he is, he can be embarrassed by such a declaration. Furthermore, many people just don't care or need to know.

Nevertheless, you *do* need to educate people who are in frequent contact with your child, or who may be in the position to give your child a meal or snack. Unfortunately, teaching others about the disease and gaining their true understanding isn't always easy. Other adults may go through a denial similar to what you experienced, and, believe it or not, some people do not accept the existence of food allergies. Given all this, prepare yourself, because mistakes *will* be made!

Be straightforward when you're talking with friends and family about your child's condition and diet, and keep your emotions in check. Your child will learn from you how *he* should educate others, so remember to be accurate, clear, and concise.

The easiest way to start educating your friends and family is to present them with a quick summary of what your child can and can't eat. You may want to give them a copy of the *Quick Start Diet Guide for Celiac Disease* in the Appendix. Go over it with the people you are talking to, and make sure they understand it thoroughly.

As you're explaining it to them, carefully watch their responses, both verbal and nonverbal. It's important to recognize whether they're really "getting it" or not. If it appears that they do not fully understand the importance of this diet to your child's well-being, try rephrasing the information to help them out.

It's important to stress the severity of getting even a tiny bit of gluten—even if you have to get overly dramatic to make your point. If they're shrugging you off, or you get the impression they're taking it too lightly, resort to using phrases such as, "Gluten is *toxic* to his system" or "Even one molecule can cause *lesions* internally." Nothing like the words "toxic" and "lesions" to make a point!

The Four Categories of Friends and Family

1. Those Who Handle It Well and "Get It"

You may be lucky enough to have a few friends or relatives who really "get it!" What a blessing. These people will really tune in when you break the news, they will ask lots of good questions, and will diligently study this book and any other information you give them. Some will even do some research on their own. When your child is planning to visit, they will stock up on gluten-free treats and will confidently plan gluten-free meals. These people are godsends to you—don't forget it, and more importantly, don't let them forget it!

2. Those Who Are Scared Even to Give Your Child a Piece of Fruit

It is important to realize that some of your friends *will* be scared of harming your child! After all, you've made the point to everyone about how serious it can be for your child to get any gluten. Some of them may be scared to death to feed him. And they may not even be aware of their own fear, much less be able to communicate it tactfully to you.

Frankly, it's okay that they're afraid—better that than to have them be too nonchalant. It's up to you to be sensitive enough to understand how they're feeling, and to help them deal with their fear, even if they haven't said anything about it. Help them overcome their anxieties by providing menu ideas, suggesting fast food restaurants and appropriate food selections, and providing foods for your child when he is with that person. But be careful not to make it *too* easy on them, or they'll never learn.

> "My best friend used to have Shari over all the time—our daughters are best friends. But now, she seems to be avoiding the opportunity to have her over, and I think it's because of Shari's diet. I'm a little angry about it, but I'm also wondering if there's something I should do?"
> —*Amy T.*

3. Those Who Think You're Exaggerating

With some conditions, a "little" of the bad stuff is okay. It's okay, for instance, for diabetics to have a little sugar; it's okay for people on low-fat diets to have a little fat. So we need to remember that many people believe "a little is okay," and may have trouble shaking that mentality.

If you're known to exaggerate about other things, it's likely that people will think you're exaggerating when you tell them your child can't have even *one molecule* of gluten. Remember the old story of the boy who cried "wolf?" Well, this is when it haunts you. Because if people think you're exaggerating, they're going to nod you off and then slip your son a cookie when you aren't looking.

"My mother-in-law absolutely refuses to have any part of a discussion about celiac disease. She thinks we're just being difficult when we explain the limitations of the diet, and has called us 'overprotective.' She has the whole family thinking we're blowing things way out of proportion and exaggerating Emily's condition. It's really frustrating."
—David L.

Be sure to let them know that you're not exaggerating or blowing things out of proportion. If you have a reputation for stretching the facts, address this issue head on. Say something like, "I know I've exaggerated about things in the past, but this is extremely important, and I hope you'll take this seriously. Every molecule of gluten will, in fact, do damage to him, and it's crucial that everyone be aware of that."

Remind everyone that "double dipping" with the knife in margarine, jelly, peanut butter, and other containers contaminates it, even if they can't *see* the crumbs, and makes it off limits to your child.

4. The "Just-Don't-Get-It" Category (Most Common)

There are actually two breeds of the Just-Don't-Get-It species. There are the "I-gotcha-say-no-more-read-ya-loud-and-clear" Just-Don't-Get-Its, and the Admittedly Acquiescent Just-Don't-Get-Its.

The "I-gotcha-say-no-more-read-ya-loud-and-clear" variety is by far the most difficult to train, because they *think* they get it. But they don't. The telltale sign that you're dealing with this breed is the nod that comes too quickly. When you say, "He can't eat gluten," the person starts nodding ferociously as though they know exactly what you're talking about (also often accompanied by a smug grin, fingers pointed at you like a cocked gun, a wink, and a clucking of the tongue). It's not necessarily that they're trying to act like they know something they don't. It's just that they may *think* they know—but they don't.

"My best friend thinks she understands the diet, and even comments to me about how easy it is. But then I find that she's been feeding Cass deli meat with modified food starch. When I called the manufacturer, it turned out the food starch is derived from wheat. I'm not mad—I realize this is a subtle and confusing part of the diet— but it's annoying because she thinks she gets it, but she doesn't."
—Tania T.

Many people *think* they get it because they assume that gluten is something more familiar than it is—for instance, that gluten is the same thing as glucose; if it's kosher, it must be okay; or if it comes from a health food store and says "natural," it has to be safe.

I'm embarrassed to admit that initially even I hung onto the hope that maybe "flour" was different from "wheat flour," and that as long as it didn't say, "wheat flour," it was okay. So these well-meaning folks *think* they're speaking our language, but they're not. Unless this is someone who spends a lot of time with your child and really needs to understand the complexities of the diet, give up. Say no more. They're a Just-Plain-Don't-Get-It, and the ferocious nodders are the toughest to teach.

The second breed of the Just-Don't-Get-It species is the Admittedly Acquiescent. These people know they're not going to get it, and they say nothing. They simply take all of the written information you give them, stack it neatly into a pile that will surely never again be touched, and listen quietly and without interruption to your "spiel." When you're finished, they offer no more than a blank stare and a vague acknowledgment that they know you were speaking and now you're finished.

Unfortunately, the Just-Don't-Get-It types are the most common. In most cases you have to just give up and pray they don't poison your child. It's best, when you have to entrust your child's meal to this type, to send something premade that can't be contaminated by utensils or dirty ovens.

How to Deal with Just-Don't-Get-It Friends and Family

Adjusting to the gluten-free lifestyle is difficult, at best. So it's understandable that you may feel resentment and anger when close friends and family fall into the Just-Don't-Get-It category. You want them to be able to support you, to help out—and instead, they make it more difficult. Not only do you have to deal with the diet without their help and understanding, but you have to watch out for the possibility that they will accidentally give your child gluten.

The fact is, they *don't* get it, and most likely, they never will. So deal with it; don't dwell on it. Give them a copy of your gluten-free products listing, and make sure you always provide them with gluten-free prepprepared meals and treats. Again, make sure your child understands his diet to the best of his ability so that he can politely refuse the cookie that Grandma sneaks him with loving intentions.

And how do you deal with Grandma? It depends on how likely she is to really understand the diet. If you think there's hope, and that her mistake was based on loving intentions, gently point out to her that she gave her beloved grandson gluten, and that you're sure she wouldn't want to cause him harm. But if she's destined to be a Just-Doesn't-Get-It for life, or if you suspect that the "accident" may have been intentional for some reason, then bite your tongue and hope that you can trust your child to make the right choice in the future.

Hiding Husbands: How to Pull Them Out of Their Caves

All husbands, as the saying goes, are not created equal. It is therefore no surprise that their responses when their child is diagnosed with celiac disease will vary.

> "When my doctor told me about Kylie's diagnosis, I turned to my husband for support; after all, I thought we were in this together. But he just shut down and won't deal with it at all – he hasn't even taken the time to learn what she can or can't eat. Now I feel even more alone than before."
> —Jenny J.

I realize that even to address this issue implies a sexist or stereotypical view of husbands/dads, and that, in fact, many husbands/dads are reading this book in order to get a better handle on how to deal with their child's condition. Those husbands, and lucky wives of those husbands, may be excused from reading this section.

But the truth is that it is usually the moms who take on the primary responsibility for the care and feeding of their children. So, it is typically the moms who are first to suspect that something's wrong, the moms who begin the often arduous and usually frustrating process of seeking medical consultation, and, ultimately, the moms who have to take principal responsibility for learning to deal with the gluten-free diet.

In our discussions with hundreds of parents who have contacted R.O.C.K. for help, we have found that most dads have a similar reaction to their child's diagnosis, and that rarely is it what Mom wants it to be. The natural reaction for many, if not most, dads is to run and hide. They don't, of course, literally run out of the room. And they may at first sound as though they're going to be very supportive—because they *want* to be supportive. But most of the time, they don't know how to start, and soon the mom has taken complete responsibility for learning the gluten-free diet.

It's important to realize that dads *want* to be involved in this diet, but may not know how to offer their support. Since moms are usually the ones who feed the kids, dads may feel that they shouldn't step in and take over that responsibility. They may ask you, "Can Natalie eat this?" Don't be tempted to answer (even if just to yourself), "Of course not, Airhead! If you were more involved with her diet, you'd know that hydrolyzed vegetable protein may have gluten in it." No, not a good response at all.

Dads love their kids just as much as moms do, and for them to recognize that they may not even know what to feed their own child can be humiliating and embarrassing. They may be scared that they will poison their own child with gluten. Rather than deal with these uncomfortable emotions, some men avoid the situation altogether, and refuse to become involved at all.

If the husband/dad in your family is making himself scarce and refusing to become involved, realize that it's up to you to give him a hand. You can help him to become more supportive and take more responsibility, which will be the ultimate win-win situation.

The first step is for you to help him learn about the gluten-free diet. The key is to teach him without him knowing that he's being taught. To "instruct" him may cause resentment and defensiveness, which will send him right back into that cave.

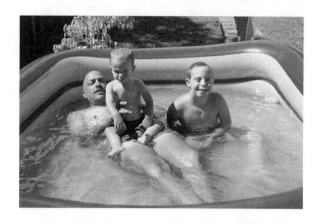

Instead, encourage him to become involved in the diet by asking him to plan a meal, or read labels at the grocery store. For some men, simply being involved in meal planning and preparation will be a new concept, not to mention the additional consideration of going gluten-free. The more he becomes involved, the more confidence he'll have in mastering the gluten-free lifestyle, and the more active role he will take in your child's diet.

Most of all, remember to be supportive and kind. You both have interesting new challenges and issues ahead, and it's important that you deal with them in a cohesive, constructive, positive manner. Most importantly, remember that you have an audience—your kids are taking note.

Relatives in Denial: It's Not My Gene!

When you talk with family members, especially the child's grandparents, you will almost certainly hear something along the lines of, "Well, he didn't get it from me!" Usually those are the same grandparents who suffer from "irritable bowel syndrome," have relatives who have had colon cancer, and find that they feel better when they avoid certain foods, such as beer or bread. But they definitely don't have celiac disease, no sirree.

The truth is that the predisposition to develop celiac disease is inherited; the genes came from someone in your child's biological family. Recent studies of relatives of people diagnosed with celiac dis-

"When Tarryn was diagnosed, it occurred to us that several people on my wife's side of the family have 'stomach problems.' Now that we know what to look for, they all seem pretty classic celiac to us. Yet not a single one will get tested. They complain about 'irritable bowel syndrome' or a 'wheat allergy,' and we try to explain that they could have celiac disease, and they should be tested. But they just won't."
—Tom B.

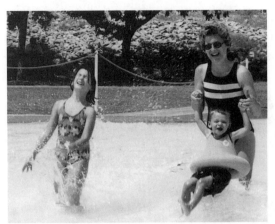

This mother and her two children have all been diagnosed with celiac disease.

ease revealed that more than 20 percent of the relatives who showed no symptoms whatsoever tested positive for celiac disease.

It is imperative that close relatives of your child with celiac disease be tested, even if there is no evidence of a disorder. The overall familial prevalence of celiac disease is estimated to be approximately 10 to 30 percent in first-degree relatives of a diagnosed celiac. First-degree relatives include the parents, siblings, and children.

You can gently remind them of the consequences to people who have celiac disease and continue to eat gluten: Research indicates that they may be 40 to 100 times more likely to develop intestinal lymphoma (cancer); they may develop a myriad of medical problems, including anemia, osteoporosis, infertility, and malnutrition; and they will likely experience gastrointestinal discomfort that they may mistakenly attribute to lactose intolerance, irritable bowel syndrome, stress, or gas.

See Chapters Twenty-One and Twenty-Two for more information on familial incidence, genetics, and testing.

Discuss It Discreetly — Remember, Kids Have Ears, Too

People will ask you about your child's condition. They're curious, and there's nothing wrong with that. Don't feel offended or intruded upon because people ask why your child is politely refusing the birthday cake or team snack. Don't whisper or act ashamed; but at the same time, you don't need to walk into a restaurant or room full of friends and declare that your child has a special diet.

Information should be distributed on a need-to-know basis. There are also varying degrees of how much information people might "need to know." Always remember that your child is listening, so be careful how you phrase the information. You need to be accurate (don't call it an allergy!). But you don't want to make it sound as if it's a burden for you, either (until your child is out of the room—then you can dump on your closest friends!).

You may want to prepare yourself early on so that you're not caught off-guard when someone asks. Depending upon the situation, the answer can be brief and factual, or lengthy and emotional. Here are a few conversation guides and some suggestions for different responses based on who you are talking to and their need-to-know rating:

- The really quick you-probably-don't-really-care-anyway-but-I-feel-I-need-to-explain response. This is best used when the waitress asks, "What? No bun on the burger?" as though you've just asked for fried worms in your salad. You could choose just to say, "That's right, he doesn't like the bun." But if you say that, chances are good that the waitress will just grab a pre-prepared burger and pluck the bun off. That's not good enough for a child with celiac disease. A better response could be, "He can't eat wheat and other things, so he can't eat the bun. It's also important that the bun never touch the burger patty." Or something equally benign that will get the point across.

- The response for acquaintances who are genuinely curious, but don't want to hear your life's story. How far you take it is best gauged by how much they seem to be "getting" as you explain it, but a good start is to say, "He has a condition called celiac disease. It requires that he be on a restricted diet—no gluten." Chances are at this point, they'll have questions: What is gluten? How did you find out he had it? Is it really rare? Will he outgrow it? Base your response from here on the questions you get.

- Friends—that's what they're there for. If you're talking with your best friend, get it off your chest. Let them know the gluten-free diet can be difficult. Frustrating. You get mad at your friends who don't get it. You get mad at your friends who have it so easy. You have enough stress in your life without having to deal with a restricted and some-times-difficult diet. When you're done, you'll feel better. Then you can get on with raising your happy, healthy gluten-free kid.

10 The Celiac-Friendly Kitchen

"I thought we were being pretty good about the diet. Then I realized we were using the same colander to drain my daughter's gluten-free pasta as we were using to drain the 'regular' pasta. How careful should we be when preparing food in the kitchen?"
—Sandra-Marie G.

You might as well face it—the days of using one knife to spread anything on toast—are toast. In fact, if you are making both gluten-containing and gluten-free peanut butter and jelly sandwiches, did you know it is a four-knife process? It's true!

Have you ever looked into someone's jelly jar? It's a sort of disgusting exercise, really, and may kill your appetite for ever eating at their house again. The point is that there are *crumbs*! Millions of gluten-containing, villi-blunting, diarrhea-inducing *crumbs* nesting comfortably in the jelly jar.

Unless your entire family is 100 percent gluten-free (and you therefore have a completely gluten-free kitchen), you need to be extremely careful about the possibility of cross-contamination. That means no sticking the knife back into the margarine container for "seconds" after spreading the first helping on toast. Any utensil that has touched gluten-containing food should not be used in the preparation of gluten-free foods. You can't stir the "regular" pasta and then use the same spoon to stir the gluten-free stuff. You can't drain the pastas in the same colander, either, unless you wash it thoroughly. When you make a grilled cheese sandwich with "regular" bread, you can't use the same pan (until you wash it thoroughly) to make a gluten-free variety.

It's not difficult to maintain a celiac-friendly kitchen, but it does take some getting used to and ongoing diligence. Make sure the entire family, even the very young kids, understand the importance of it.

Tips for Keeping a Celiac-Friendly Kitchen

Spreadables

- **Learn to do the "Gob Drop."** No, it's not a new dance, nor a new candy. It's a method of scooping up a gob of margarine (or peanut butter, jelly, mayonnaise, or any other spread), and dropping it onto your slice of bread (or pancake—you get the idea). The key to a good gob drop is learning how *much* of a gob to grab. The beauty of the gob drop is that because the knife has not actually touched the bread, it's okay to reinsert it and go for another gob! But once you've used the knife to spread your gob, you cannot go back for more. So why does it take four knives to make a peanut butter and jelly sandwich? Well, just imagine you're making two PB&Js: one with "regular" bread, and one with your really-delicious-because-you've-perfected-the-recipe gluten-free bread. Assume that you're using gluten-free peanut butter and jelly for both sandwiches. You start with the gluten-containing sandwich, and you use knife number-one for the peanut butter. After a carefully measured gob-drop, you are now ready to spread. But after the knife has touched the bread, it can no longer be used for *anything*! Not more peanut butter, not jelly—not *even* to finish making the "regular" sandwich! Because when that knife goes back into the jar, it is laden with gluten. You repeat the process with jelly, and before you know it, you've used several knives for just a couple of sandwiches!

  Do you need to do the gob drop if you're dropping onto a gluten-free piece of bread (pancake, etc.)? You should. While the gluten-free crumbs won't cause a problem in terms of gluten contamination, they could cause you to stop and wonder whether the crumbs are gluten-containing or gluten-free. We have thrown away more than a few jars of mayonnaise because we didn't know for sure.

- **Buy separate "spreadables."** As an alternative to doing the "gob drop," you can keep separate containers for things that are easily contaminated, such as margarine, cream cheese, and jelly. It's safest to have separate containers, even if the margarine you use is GF. Mark the containers "GF only," and make sure they're used only for gluten-free food preparation.

Utensils

- **Have separate colanders.** Pasta leaves a residue, and is therefore very difficult to remove completely. It's a good idea to have separate colanders: one for gluten-free pastas, and one for gluten-containing pastas. (Of course you could drain the gluten-free pasta first, and make sure you wash it thoroughly after you drain gluten-containing pasta in it.) Because we make two types of pasta on spaghetti night—one with gluten and one without—it's easiest to make them at the same time and use two separate colanders. If you have more than one, it's a good idea to dedicate one of them to the gluten-free pastas, and then mark them with a permanent marker so that there will never be any question which colander is used for which type of pasta.

- **It goes both ways.** When separating utensils and other items used in the kitchen, remember that it's just as important to keep gluten-free foods *out* of the "gluten-only" containers as it is to keep gluten-containing foods out of the gluten-free containers. In other words, it's obvious that you don't want to put gluten-containing pasta into a gluten-free colander. But sometimes people forget that putting gluten-free pasta into a colander dedicated for "regular" pasta is just as bad! The gluten residue on the colander contaminates the gluten-free pasta, defeating the purpose of separating the utensils in the first place.

- **Use lots of aluminum foil.** To ensure that gluten-free food remains uncontaminated, use aluminum foil for any cooking you do on a cookie sheet, or any other surface, for that matter. If you prefer to cook directly on the sheet, make sure you designate one for gluten-free purposes, keep it in a separate area, if possible, and never use it with gluten-containing food.

Making and Toasting Bread

- **Buy a breadmaker.** Even if you love to bake, I suggest buying a breadmaker, because you will be making a lot of bread and it will make your life easier when you're out of time and energy. You will need to do some research to find one that can accommodate the heavy gluten-free dough. Look for the models with the greatest horsepower and large mixing paddles. (I'm not saying it's absolutely *necessary* to buy a breadmaker. Many mixes turn out well without one, and the bakers amongst you may not need one either. But breadmakers can help if you're short on time, or if the kids make their own bread.)

- **While you're at it, buy a bread slicer.** Bread slicers can be found near the breadmakers at most stores that carry household items.

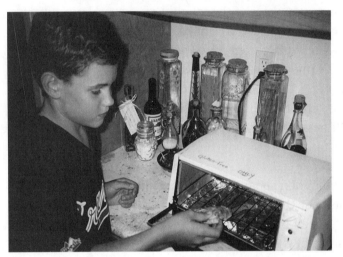

The loaf of bread fits inside the slicer, which has slits every ¾" or so. The slicer comes with an electric knife, which you insert into the slits as you cut. It slices the bread in even slices and makes it look just like "regular" bread. As you know, how it *looks* is every bit as important as how it *tastes* to a child!

It's important to have two toaster ovens, one of which should be clearly marked "Gluten-Free Only."

- **Have separate toasters or toaster ovens.** Once a "regular" piece of bread touches the grill of a toaster or toaster oven, the grill is contaminated, and you should not use that same toaster or toaster oven for gluten-free bread (unless everyone in your family is very good about wiping off the toaster after gluten-containing bread has been used). If you have a four-slice toaster, you may be tempted to dedicate two of the slots for gluten-free bread, leaving the other two slots for "regular" bread. Don't do it. Anyone who has wiped up around a toaster knows that toast practically *throws* crumbs around. There is almost no way to pull a piece of "regular" bread out of one slot without dropping crumbs into another slot. There's really no way around it unless your kitchen is 100 percent gluten-free—you need separate toasters. Forget aesthetics and get out that permanent marker, clearly marking one "gluten-free" and the other "gluten only." That way even guests won't make a mistake.

Food Preparation

- **Clean those crumbs!** Remember to wipe up bread crumbs and other gluten-containing messes. All it takes is for someone to set a gluten-free sandwich on a plate that had a gluten-containing item on it, and the whole point of eating that gluten-free sandwich is for naught.

- **Get in the habit of making the gluten-free version first.** If you're making a grilled cheese sandwich, make the gluten-free version first. That way you can use the same pan (assuming it has a good non-stick finish and you clean it well) for both the gluten-free and the "regular" versions. While you're getting into new habits, you might as well get used to making more of the gluten-free version than you think you'll need. Otherwise, just as you finish cooking the heavily-laden gluten sandwich, your child with celiac disease will change her mind and decide that yes, she does in fact want another one. And then you get to wash the pan *two* more times!

- **Order mixes.** Throughout this book, we try to emphasize that you can avoid specialty stores, doing most of your shopping at a "regular" grocery store. However, there are some products that are best to buy either over the Internet or via direct mail. (See the Resource Guide for companies that carry mixes you can send away for.) These include mixes for bread, pizza dough crust, pancakes, cakes, cookies, brownies, and muffins. You'll appreciate that stash of cake mixes when you suddenly realize that one of your child's classmates is having a birthday party at school!

- **Be creative.** Get in the habit of thinking, "How can I make that gluten-free" when you see a delicious recipe or meal. There are suggestions for being especially creative in Chapter Twelve.

Food Storage

- **Try to separate the gluten-free foods in the pantry and refrigerator.** By dedicating shelves or drawers to gluten-free products, you accomplish a few things. You decrease the chance that a guest or babysitter will accidentally give your child something with gluten. In addition, if guests or babysitters have questions about whether or not a food is safe, by having gluten-free foods in designated areas, you eliminate any question. You also create the sense that there are lots of things your child can eat. Sometimes when they look in a pantry, they tend to see so many foods that they *can't* have, that they have trouble seeing the things they *can* eat. This can be really dis-heartening for them. But when they see shelves loaded with gluten-free items—even if they're not treats, but just mixes, pasta, and other "staples"—they realize that there are many things they can eat.

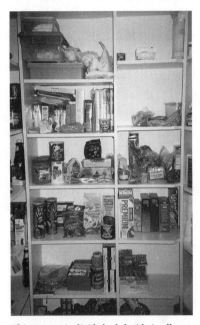

This pantry is divided—left side is all gluten-free food; right side is not gluten free. It's important to have a lot of food on the gluten-free side so the kids see that they have plenty of snacks.

- **Make a special "GF Treats" area.** Keep a drawer or cupboard that is designated especially for your gluten-free child, and make sure it's filled with all sorts of great treats. It's important to have an area that she sees *filled* with fun foods that she can eat—even if you have to make her wait until after dinner! It's not enough just to have the treats on hand, mixed with all the other gluten-containing treats. Kids tend to look at the entire picture, and see "nothing" that they can eat.

- **Buy small, brightly colored removable labels.** These work well for sticking on plastic ware used to store leftovers. You can write your child's name or just "GF" on the label, or simply have a designated "GF color" for food containers. (If other people use your kitchen and feed your kids, a "GF color" may not be clear enough. If that's the case, you should write your child's name or "GF" on the label.)

When Guests Visit

Okay, so you've finally gotten the routine down, and even your two-year-old has perfected the gob drop. But now you have a houseful of guests coming for Thanksgiving. At our house, it's a "mi casa es su casa" environment. We frequently have people staying with us, and they're encouraged to help themselves to anything in the fridge.

Accommodating, yes. But visiting guests who help themselves to the fridge will be your greatest challenge in keeping a celiac-friendly kitchen.

If the guests are "regulars," it's important to initially explain in detail how critical it is to keep the kitchen celiac-friendly. Chances are they are already well aware of your child's condition, but the extent of their understanding will vary,

Do You Need to Keep a Gluten-Free Bathroom Too?

Shampoos and Lotions: I have become so accustomed to reading labels that I find myself reading ingredients on nonfood items. It was in the shower that I realized that nearly every shampoo we use contains wheat! Many people have asked whether this can cause a reaction in someone with celiac disease. In other words, can gluten be absorbed through the skin? No. According to John Zone, M.D., a dermatologist who is an expert on dermatitis herpetiformis (sister condition to celiac disease that manifests itself on the skin), gluten that is present in topically applied make-ups and lotions is not absorbed, because the protein molecules in gluten are too large.*

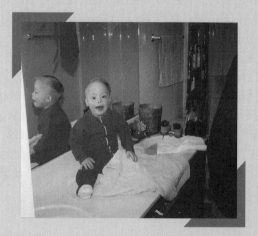

Toothpaste: Toothpaste is supposed to be used in miniscule amounts, and, of course, spat out. But kids often smear a gob of toothpaste the size of a Tootsie Roll on their toothbrush, and if it tastes good enough, they'll swallow it and go for seconds. Most toothpastes are gluten free, but it's a good idea to check with the manufacturer to make sure there aren't any hidden sources of gluten.

Vitamins: Some doctors will tell you that if your child has a healthy diet, regardless of whether or not she has celiac disease, she does not need vitamins. Others are adamant that supplements are an important part of a child's diet. If you are giving your child vitamins, check for fillers, stabilizers, starch, and flavorings. These things may contain gluten, and should be clarified with the manufacturer.

---

* *Gluten-Free Living Magazine*, March/April 1999.

depending upon whose friend it is, how old they are, and how tuned-in they are to the situation. Whether they understand or not, it is crucial to teach all guests that there is never any double-dipping in the spreadables. If your toasters and utensils are well-marked, it should be clear what can and can't be used for food preparation, but call it to their attention in the beginning, just in case. You'll have to watch closely at first, and even years later you'll find your blood pressure increases every time guests are cooking in your kitchen.

If the guests are not regulars, you need to decide how much information to give them. Gauge their interest level, their ability to thoroughly understand, how long they're staying, and how likely they are to use the kitchen. One helpful trick is to buy small tubs of the spreadables your child is most likely to need for the duration of the visit—margarine, peanut butter, cream cheese, mayo. Mark her containers clearly with her name followed by the word "ONLY!" and threatening pictures of what will happen to anyone else who uses it. Make sure that your child eats only from those containers during the visit.

Try to teach your visitors the gob drop. Some will get it, but some just can't resist sticking the knife back into the container. Work with them, and try to educate them in a firm but friendly way, but remember to use the dedicated gluten-free spreadables for your child. When the guests have gone, the safest option is to toss the "community containers" and start fresh.

Most of the time, you'll find it's easier just to do all the meal preparation and serving yourself. But don't fall into that trap. Guests *like* to help, and you don't want to make them feel awkward. Give them something to do that won't involve a risk of cross-contamination. Have them wash the veggies or slice the meat, and prepare yourself for the fact that there probably will be mistakes, and that life will go on.

11 Shopping
Is There More to Life Than Fritos?

"Off I went—boldly going where it seemed no one else had ever gone—my first shopping trip in search of gluten-free goodies. My son was begging for crackers, so I started in the cracker aisle, trying to find one without gluten. You know, not one single package had "gluten" in the ingredients. I was delighted! What a breeze this was going to be!"
—Danna Korn

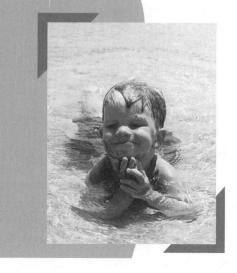

When Tyler was first diagnosed with celiac disease, our doctor, trying to be upbeat, nonchalantly explained that this would mean that we would just need to modify our diets, and that we would need to eliminate—you may want to write this down, he suggested—wheat, oats, rye, and barley, which we're all supposed to know is what they use to make malt. Oh, and anything else that may contain gluten.

Hmmm. That really didn't sound too tough. After all, we were well-educated people—how hard could it be to cut out five ingredients? As I checked out of the doctor's office, they suggested I see the hospital dietitian, who had a list of gluten-free foods and forbidden ingredients. I figured it wouldn't hurt to have a little help, so I dropped by, figuring I was her forty-third celiac mom that month, and asked her for the gluten-free foods list.

The five seconds it took her to register my request in her brain should have been my first clue that the folks at the hospital didn't come across this often. My second clue should have been that she had to dig through several folders before she finally pulled out a well-worn and obviously long-forgotten blue sheet that said, "Gluten-Free Forbidden Ingredients."

I nearly choked when I saw the size-four font that literally filled the entire page with things my son could *not* have! There was even a back side! What happened to just wheat, oats, rye, barley, and malt? "Oh," she explained, "gluten is in all sorts of ingredients you wouldn't normally think of," and she started to read to me off the sheet. I grumpily snatched it away from her. I can read myself, thank you very much.

After pulling myself together and remembering that my bloated-belly toddler needed me to be strong for him, I armed myself with the blue sheet of forbidden ingredients, and headed to my neighborhood grocery store.

My son was begging for crackers, so I started in the cracker aisle, trying to find one without gluten. Hmmm. You know, not one single package had "gluten" in the ingredients. I was delighted! What a breeze this was going to be! But then I checked my list again—"flour." My heart sunk. Could it possibly be by some grace of God that *flour* is different from *wheat flour*? After all, the ingredients label doesn't *say* "wheat flour," it just says "flour." It was hopeful and naïve thinking, I knew.

On with the search for a cracker that Tyler could eat. It only takes a few hours of dealing with the gluten-free diet to know there's no point even in going *down* the cracker aisle, but I was in my infancy of gluten-free(dom), and thought maybe some of the "rice crackers" would be okay. Flour in everything. I gave up and headed to the bread aisle. Nothing.

By now we were well into the second hour of "shopping," with a completely empty cart. My son and I were both crying—he because he was hungry and bored, and I because I couldn't have been sadder or more frustrated. And this was only the beginning.

As we started to leave, I passed through the chips aisle and happened to pick up a bag of Fritos. What? No flour? I checked the huge list of forbidden additives, and none were found in the ingredients listing on this precious bag of Fritos! My sadness turned to relief and gratitude to the Frito-Lay company. I grabbed four bags and headed for the check-out stand. Thank God for Fritos.

Can You Ever Do Most of Your Shopping at a "Regular" Grocery Store Again?

Many parents with newly diagnosed kids fear that they will have to do all of their shopping in expensive and inconvenient health food stores. Well, stop worrying about taking out that third mortgage just to pay the food bill. Because you *can* do most of your shopping at a "regular" grocery store, and it's really not that hard to do, once you figure out a family menu plan that works for you. You can even buy generic foods, if you put a little effort into it. Yes, you will still need to head to a health food store and maybe buy some things by mail order, but 95 percent of your shopping can be done at your neighborhood grocery store.

> *"I figure my days of shopping at the local grocery store are history. I'm assuming I'll have to do all of my shopping at a health food store or by mail—that's so expensive and inconvenient!"*
> —Charlanne O.

Start by stocking up on gluten-free staples. Some will be more expensive, but the peace of mind is well worth the money. Some brands of the following staple items contain gluten, and others don't. In fact, there are many staples that rarely, if ever, contain gluten. But even for those that usually do contain gluten (i.e., soy sauce), with a little homework (calls to manufacturers, label reading, and/or gluten-free shopping guides), it's easy to find the following "staple items" in any major grocery chain:

- mayonnaise
- ketchup
- mustard
- gluten-free soy sauce
- gluten-free teriyaki sauce
- salad dressings
- margarine/butter
- sugar
- brown sugar
- corn starch
- nonstick sprays
- yogurt
- milk
- hot cocoa
- marshmallows
- cheese
- chili
- chicken stock
- soups
- bouillon

Develop a List of Safe Products Your Child Likes

- **Create or buy a product listing of gluten-free foods.** Keep it neatly organized so that when you need the information, it's there. You may even want to have two copies, each in a three-ring binder. You can keep one in the pantry and one in the car (so that you can check on particular products if you're at the grocery store or a restaurant and the need arises). If you want to generate your own list, give yourself a head start by going to the product listings at celiac disease web sites. There are some phenomenal sites now! And remember, just because an item is *not* on a published gluten-free list does *not* mean it has gluten in it. Keep digging to be sure. See the Resource Guide at the back of this book for a listing of manufacturers and distributors.

- **Date your products list.** Whether you make your own list as a result of calls to manufacturers or are using lists received from companies, date them! Ingredients change, and you should check frequently to make sure the products are still gluten-free.

Keeping Your Medicine Cabinet Safely Stocked

Usually it's not until your child has a fever of 104 degrees at 2 a.m. on a Saturday that you realize you have no idea which medications are gluten-free. Many contain starch, fillers, stabilizers, flavorings, or other ingredients that could contain gluten. Be sure to call the major brand-name companies to find out which cold medications, fever reducers, analgesics, and cough medicines are gluten-free.

The Resource Guide in this book has contact information for companies that have gluten-free medication databases or websites, or that sell guides for gluten-free medications.

- **Call manufacturers.** Get in the habit of calling every toll-free number you can find on the side of a box. It doesn't matter whether the product appears to be gluten-free or not—it can be a box of saltines, for that matter. But call to ask if they have a list of their gluten-free products. You'll be pleasantly surprised at how many food distributors and manufacturers are very knowledgeable about gluten.

- **Get out that permanent marker.** It's a good idea to mark "GF" in permanent marker directly on the product labels when you learn they're gluten-free. This will avoid any questions, especially if other people are feeding your kids.

- **Save labels of safe foods for a month or two.** In the beginning, before you're *really* organized, it can be very helpful to save the labels of products that you discover are gluten-free. Keep them in a large zip-seal bag, and take them to the grocery store with you, just in case you have trouble remembering which items are safe. Of course, after a few months the safe products will be etched in your brain!

Beware of "New and Improved"

Many consumers get excited when they see the words "new and improved." Sure, it's usually just a marketing gimmick, but for people with celiac disease everywhere, "new and improved" means "start from scratch" in ensuring that it's gluten-free. That trusty brand of gluten-free mayo may not be so gluten-free anymore.

Even without label changes, remember that just because a product is gluten-free today doesn't mean that it will be gluten-free tomorrow. Check labels frequently for ingredient changes, and call the manufacturers often to make sure that their sources and ingredients are still gluten-free.

Buying Generics

Yes, it's even possible to buy gluten-free generic products. The first thing to do is contact the corporate headquarters for the chain of stores you prefer, and ask if they have a list of their gluten-free products. Chances are they won't, but it's worth a try. Some major grocery chains even have a list of their generic gluten-free products on the Internet.

If your preferred stores don't have a list, you can dig a little to find the generics that are gluten-free. Start small, and be prepared. Pick four or five generic foods that you want to check into—maybe things that you want your child to eat or that were favorites before a diagnosis. Buy them, even not knowing whether or not they're gluten-free, and have them in front of you before you call. Call the corporate headquarters and work your way to their head nutritionist. It's not always easy to find that person, but persevere, and you will get there.

Be nice! This person can be your very best friend, or can be lazy and give you the dreaded, "I don't know." But if you say that you realize you are asking a lot, but could they help you determine whether or not some of the foods are gluten-free, chances are they'll be receptive and cooperative.

Unfortunately, you can't just ask if the products are gluten-free. Focus on the ingredients that are suspect—modified food starch, for instance. Ask if they can find out what the source is: wheat, corn, or another source. Usually they know that information right away. Go through all of the suspect ingredients until you have determined that the product is or is not gluten-free. Make note of it, keep it in your binder, and be sure to check back often because ingredients, as you know, change.

Avoiding Hidden Sources of Gluten

Some ingredients listed on labels *may* contain gluten—or they may not. It depends upon the source of the ingredient in question. For instance, modified food starch may be derived from corn, in which case it is okay, or from wheat, in which case it is of course not gluten-free.

A list of safe and forbidden ingredients and additives is provided on pages 62-66, courtesy of www.celiac.com. Keep it posted in a kitchen cabinet, or where you'll remember it in your three-ring binder.

Safe and Forbidden Ingredients and Additives

(courtesy of www.celiac.com, 9-00)

Safe List

Acacia Gum
Acorn Quercus
Alcohol (Spirits—Specific Types)
Adzuki Bean
Agar
Almond Nut
Amaranth
Annatto
Apple Cider Vinegar
Arabic Gum
Arrowroot
Artichokes
Astragalus Gummifer
Balsamic Vinegar
Beans
Bean, Adzuki
Bean, Hyacinth
Bean, Lentil
Bean, Mung
Bean Romano (Chickpea)
Bean Tepary
Besan
Bicarbonate of Soda (some contain
   gluten)
Buckwheat
Butter (beware of additives)
Carageenan Chondrus Crispus
Carob Bean
Carob Bean Gum
Carob Flour
Cassava Manihot Esculenta
Cellulose*
Cellulose Gum
Cheeses (except blue & chilton)
Chickpea

Corn
Corn Flour
Corn Meal
Cornstarch
Cowitch
Cowpea
Cream of Tartar
Eggs
Fish (fresh)
Flaked Rice
Flax
Fruit (including dried)
Gelatin
Gram flour (chick peas)
Grits, Corn
Guar Gum
Herbs
Hyacinth Bean
Job's Tears
Kasha (roasted buckwheat)
Kudzu Root Starch
Lentil
Locust Bean Gum
Maize
Maize Waxy
Maltodextrin****
Manioc
Masa Flour
Masa Harina
Meat (fresh)
Methyl Cellulose**
Milk
Millet
Milo
Mung Bean

Nut, Acorn
Nut, Almond
Oats***
Oils and Fats
Peas
Pea—Chick
Pea—Cow
Pea Flour
Pigeon Peas
Polenta
Potatoes
Potato Flour
Prinus
Psyllium
Quinoa
Ragi
Rape
Rice
Rice Flour
Rice Vinegar
Romano Bean (chickpea)
Sago Flour
Sago Palm
Saifun (bean threads)
Seed—Sesame
Seed—Sunflower
Soba (be sure it's 100% buckwheat)
Sorghum
Sorghum Flour

Soy
Soybean
Spices (pure)
Spirits (Specific Types)
Starch (made in USA)
Sunflower Seed
Sweet Chestnut Flour
Tapioca
Tapioca Flour
Teff
Teff Flour
Tepary Bean
Tofu-Soya Curd
Tragacanth
Tragacanth Gum
Turmeric (Kurkuma)
Urad Beans
Urad Dal (peas) Vegetables
Urid flour
Vinegars (Specific Types)
Waxy Maize
Whey
Wild Rice
Wines
Wine Vinegars (& Balsamic)
Xanthan Gum
Yam Flour
Yogurt

*Cellulose is a carbohydrate polymer of D-glucose. It is the structural material of plants, such as wood in trees. It contains no gluten protein.

**Methyl cellulose is a chemically modified form of cellulose that makes a good substitute for gluten in rice-based breads, etc.

***Cross-contamination with wheat is a slight possibility.

****Maltodextrin is prepared as a white powder or concentrated solution by partial hydrolysis of corn starch or potato starch with safe and suitable acids and enzymes. (1) Maltodextrin, when listed on food sold in the USA, must be (per FDA regulation) made from corn or potato. This rule does NOT apply to vitamin or mineral supplements and medications. (2) Donald Kasarda, Ph.D., a research chemist specializing on grain proteins, of the United States Department of Agriculture, found that all maltodextrins in the USA are made from corn starch, using enzymes that are NOT derived from wheat, rye, barley, or oats. On that basis he believes that celiacs need not be too concerned about maltodextrins, though he cautions that there is no guarantee that a manufacturer won't change their process to use wheat starch or a gluten-based enzyme in the future.

Safe Additives

Acacia Gum
Adipic Acid
Annatto Color
Arabic Gum
Ascorbic Acid
Aspartame (can cause IBS symptoms)
BHA
BHT
Beta Carotene
Biotin
Calcium Chloride
Calcium Phosphate
Carboxymethylcellulose
Carob Bean Gum
Carrageenan
Cellulose Gum
Cetyl Alcohol
Citric Acid (made in USA)*
Corn Swetener
Corn Syrup Solids
Demineralized Whey
Dextrimaltose
Dextrose
Dioctyl Sodium
Folic Acid—Folacin
Fructose
Fumaric Acid
Glutamic Acid
Glutamine (amino acid)
Glycerol Monooleate
Guar Gum
Invert Sugar
Lactic Acid
Lactose
Lecithin
Locust Bean Gum

Magnesium Hydroxide
Malic Acid
Microcrystalline Cellulose
Modified Food Starch (made in USA)
MSG (made in USA)
M Vitamins & Minerals
Niacin-Niacinamide
Polyglycerol
Polysorbate 60; 80
Potassium Citrate
Potassium Iodide
Propylene Glycol Monostearete
Propylgallate
Pyridoxine Hydrochloride
Sodium Acid Pyraphosphate
Sodium Ascorbate
Sodium Benzoate
Sodium Citrate
Sodium Hexametaphosphate
Sodium Nitrate
Sodium Silaco Aluminate
Sorbitol-Mannitol (can cause IBS symptoms)
Sphingolipids
Sucrose
Sulfosuccinate
Tartaric Acid
TBHQ is Tetra or Tributylhydroquinone
Thiamine Hydrochoride
Tragacanth Gum
Tri-Calcium Phosphate
Vanillan
Vitamin A (palmitate)
Xanthan Gum

*Citric Acid: All the citric acid produced in the US is made from corn. Outside the USA the acid can also be derived from other sources of dextrose, including cane sugar and wheat. Some of the citric acid used in the US is imported from other countries, such as China. Imported citric acid may be made from corn, sugar, or wheat. USA made citric acid capacity remains stable. There are three domestic producers of citric acid—Archer Daniels Midland, Cargill, and Haarmann & Reimer—with total capability of 460 million lb/yr of citric acid. All three produce citric acid through the fermentation of corn-based dextrose.

Forbidden List

Abyssinian Hard
  (Wheat Triticum duran)
Alcohol (Spirits—Specific Types)
Baking Soda ****
Barley Hordeum vulgare
Barley Malt
Beer
Blue Cheese (made with bread)
Bran
Bread Flour
Brown Flour
Bulgur (Bulgur Wheat/Nuts)
Bulgur Wheat
Calcium Caseinate (Contains MSG)
Caramel Color***
Cereal Binding
Chilton
Citric Acid (made outside USA)
Couscous
Dextrins*
Durum Wheat Triticum
Edible Starch
Einkorn Wheat
Farina Graham
Filler
Fu (dried wheat gluten)
Germ
Glutamate (Free)
Graham Flour
Granary Flour
Gravy Cubes ****
Groats (barley, buckwheat, or oats)
Ground Spices ****
Gum Base
Hydrolyzed Plant Protein (HPP)
Hydrolyzed Vegetable Protein (HVP)
Kamut (Pasta wheat)
Malt
Malt Extract
Malt Flavoring

Malt Syrup
Malt Vinegar
Matzo Semolina
Miso****
Modified Food Starch****
  (made outside USA)
Mono and Diglycerides**
MSG (Made outside USA)****
Mustard Powder ****
Nuts, Wheat Oats Avena stativa
Pasta
Pearl Barley
Rice Malt (contains barley or Koji)
Rye
Scotch Whisky
Semolina
Semolina Triticum
Shoyu (soy sauce)****
Small Spelt
Soba Noodles****
Sodium Caseinate (Contains MSG)
Soy Sauce
Spirits (Specific Types)
Spelt Triticum spelta
Starch (outside USA)
Stock Cubes****
Strong Flour
Suet in Packets
Tabbouleh
Teriyaki Sauce
Triticale X triticosecale
Udon (wheat noodles)
Vegetable Starch
Vinegars (Specific Types)
Vitamins ****
Wheat, Abyssinian
Wheat Triticum aestivum
Wheat Nuts
Hard triticum durum
Hard Wheat

(Continued on next page.)

Wheat, Bulgur

Wheat Durum Triticum

Wheat Germ

Wheat Triticum mononoccum

Wheat Starch*****

White Vinegar (problem for some)

Whole-Meal Flour

Dextrin is an incompletely hydrolyzed starch. It is prepared by dry heating corn, waxy maize, waxy milo, potato, arrowroot, WHEAT, rice, tapioca, or sago starches, or by dry heating the starches after: (1) Treatment with safe and suitable alkalis, acids, or pH control agents and (2) drying the acid or alkali treated starch. (1) Therefore, unless you know the source, you must avoid dextrin. - May 1997 Sprue-Nik News.(1) Federal Register (4-1-96 Edition) 21CFR Ch.1, Section 184.12277. (2) Federal Register (4-1-96) 21 CFR. Ch.1, Section 184.1444

** Mono and diglycerides can contain a wheat carrier in the USA. While they are derivatives of fats, carbohydrate chains may be used as a binding substance in their preparation, which are usually corn or wheat, so this needs to be checked out with the manufacturer.*

*** The problem with caramel color is it may or may not contain gluten, depending on how it is manufactured. In the USA caramel color must conform with the FDA standard of identity from 21CFR CH.1. This statute says: "the color additive caramel is the dark-brown liquid or solid material resulting from the carefully controlled heat treatment of the following food-grade carbohydrates: Dextrose (corn sugar), Invert sugar, Lactose (milk sugar), Malt syrup (usually from barley malt), Molasses (from cane), Starch Hydrolysates and fractions thereof (can include wheat), Sucrose (cane or beet)." Also, acids, alkalis, and salts are listed as additives which may be employed to assist the caramelization process.*

****Can utilize a gluten-containing grain or by-product in the manufacturing process, or as an ingredient.*

***** Most celiac organizations in the USA and Canada do not believe that wheat starch is safe for celiacs. In Europe, however, Codex Alimentarius Quality wheat starch is considered acceptable in the celiac diet by most doctors and celiac organizations. This is a higher quality of wheat starch than is generally available in the USA or Canada.*

Additional Things to Beware Of

- Rice and soy beverages (i.e., Rice Dream), because their production process utilizes barley enzymes.
- Bad advice from health-food store employees (i.e., that spelt and/or kamut is/are safe for celiacs).
- Cross-contamination between food store bins selling raw flours and grains (usually via the scoops).
- Wheat-bread crumbs in butter, jams, toaster, counter, etc.
- Lotions, creams, and cosmetics (for those with dermatitis herpetaformis).
- Stamps, envelopes, or other gummed labels.
- Toothpaste and mouthwash.
- Medicines: many contain gluten.
- Cereals: most contain malt flavoring, or some other non-GF ingredient.
- Some brands of rice paper.
- Sauce mixes and sauces (soy sauce, fish sauce, catsup, mustard, mayonnaise, etc.).
- Ice cream.
- Packet & canned soups.
- Dried meals and gravy mixes.
- Laxatives.
- Grilled restaurant food—gluten contaminated grill.
- Fried restaurant foods—gluten contaminated grease.
- Ground spices—wheat flour is commonly used to prevent clumping.

Menu Planning

One of the most important things to do if you want to shop at a "regular" grocery store is to figure out several meals that your entire family enjoyed pre-diagnosis, and revise them to be gluten-free. For instance, if your family enjoys burritos made with flour tortillas, improvise with corn tortillas. If your family likes ranch dressing but the dressing you use has gluten in it, find one that is gluten-free and switch. The next chapter will specifically outline suggested menu ideas.

Be sure to plan ahead. Before shopping, make sure you know what meals you want to prepare that week, so that you can make calls to manufacturers *before* you go to the store.

Shopping at Health Food Stores or by Mail Order and Online

There are some staple gluten-free items that are good to have on hand, and that are only available by mail order, or in a health food store. These days, they all taste incredible! You almost can't go wrong with the wonderful mixes available today by Internet and phone. It's a good idea to stock up on them, so that when you need them they're there. These items include:

- Bread mix (to be made with or without a breadmaker)
- Pizza dough crust mix and ready-made pizza crusts
- Pasta (all different shapes; kids love to have a variety)
- Mixes for cookies, muffins, brownies, cakes
- Pancake/waffle mix
- Ready-to-eat snacks, such as ice cream cones and pretzels

Don't feel guilty about using mixes rather than baking from scratch. Ingredients for gluten-free baked goods, such as xanthan gum and the variety of different flours used, are very expensive. The cost usually turns out to be the same or even less (especially if you count all the really gross batches of breads and cookies you'll have to throw away if you're experimenting on your own) when you use mixes.

Another great thing about mixes is that they're easy enough for some kids to make themselves at an early age (or, with some adult supervision). Remember, keeping the kids involved in their food selection and preparation gives them a sense of control, and helps them feel good about their diet.

The best reason to stock up on and use mixes is that the mixes have come a *long* way! When our son was first diagnosed, there weren't any (at least that we knew of) mixes that we could buy for baked goods, so we had to make our baked goods from scratch. Once, when he was three, I worked all day in the kitchen perfecting a chocolate chip cookie recipe to the point where I thought it was just about palatable. I felt like Beaver Cleaver's mom, and was *so* excited to be able to offer Tyler and his three-year-old buddy, A.J., some cookies, fresh from the oven— an act most moms take for granted. Beaming, I set the plate in front of them and watched carefully for their reactions. Tyler took his cookie first. His eyes lit up, and he said, "Yummy cookie, Mommy!" A.J. ran for the nearest trash can and spat for a good five minutes.

If you prefer to grind your own rice flour and bake from scratch, you have my respect and admiration. But if you're limited on time, or just don't have the desire to bake from scratch every time, give the mixes a try. (See the Resource Guide at the end of this book for a listing of places to send away for mixes.)

Get Used to Stocking Up

Because there are *some* items that need to be purchased through direct mail, the Internet, or health food stores, it's a good idea to stock up on those items. It's also a good idea to stock up on "favorites" when you encounter them. Especially good brands or flavors of cereal, crackers, pasta, mixes, pretzels, and other difficult-to-find items are welcome sights in the pantry when you're caught short on menu ideas.

12

The Chapter You've Been Waiting For

Menu and Snack Ideas!

"Hunter really misses chicken fingers, fish sticks, corn dogs, and other things he can't have anymore. I'm really not much of a cook and can't figure out how to make these things without gluten."
—Danielle V.

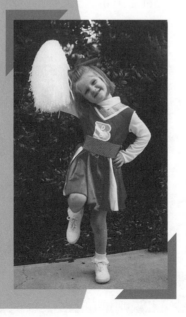

There are several excellent cookbooks on the market that are loaded with wonderful gluten-free recipes, so I am not going to provide recipes for difficult-to-make gourmet fare. Many of the recipes for baked goods that you'll find in gluten-free cookbooks require rice, tapioca, potato, or other gluten-free flours, and other ingredients you may not usually use such as xanthan gum. And having tried a number of those recipes, I can tell you that they are delicious, and you most definitely will want some of those cookbooks on hand.

But there are plenty of times when you just don't want to have to mix a bunch of flours, or pay ludicrous amounts of money for ingredients such as xanthan gum. That's what this chapter is about—learning to be a creative cook in a gluten-free sort of way.

This chapter will spark some ideas so that you can put together quick snacks and easy meals that your child will enjoy. Because they're simple, commonsense ideas, you'll be able to modify dishes that your entire family enjoys quickly and easily.

Getting Creative Is Easy!

The most important thing about cooking from now on is to *be creative*. Don't despair, thinking that your child will never again enjoy chicken nuggets. Grab some gluten-free flour—it really doesn't matter what kind—and roll the chicken in it. A bunch of oil and a big mess later, you have chicken nuggets! Thought doughnuts were a thing of the past? Nope. Buy a doughnut maker, use any gluten-free muffin or cake mix you have lying around, and voila! Doughnuts! Need a pie crust? Crush some gluten-free cookies, add some margarine, and push it into a pie tin. Really, almost anything can be modified to be gluten-free, and usually it's not too tough to do so. (The exceptions are for breads, homemade pastas, cookies, cakes, and muffins. You'll be most successful using a mix or a gluten-free recipe for these.)

If you want to make an old family favorite but it isn't gluten-free, work with it. To illustrate how easy it is to adapt a recipe to be gluten-free, I opened a cookbook (*Weight Watchers Quick Meals*) and landed on a page with a recipe for Crunchy Garlic-Broiled Halibut. Ingredients include parsley, olive oil, garlic cloves, halibut steaks, and bread crumbs. Substitute crunched-up potato chips for the bread crumbs, and you have yourself a gluten-free version that probably tastes even better than the original.

Feel like making a fancy gourmet dish like chicken cordon bleu? Take chicken breasts, flatten them out (you may want to pound them to make them more

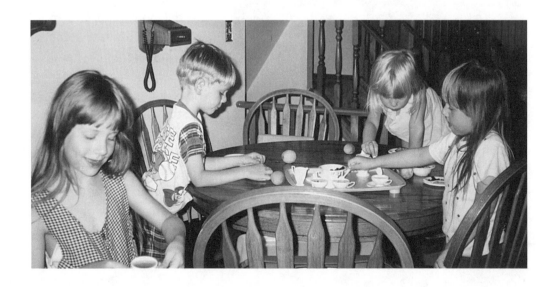

Homemade "Hamburger Helper"

With a little experimentation, you can come up with recipes for convenience foods your child craves. For example, here is a homemade version of "Hamburger Helper" that is almost as hassle free as the name brand.

- Cook 1 lb. hamburger. Drain fat.
- Add taco seasoning packet (many brands available in grocery stores are gluten-free).
- In a separate pot, boil about two cups gluten-free pasta (elbows or fun shapes are best). Drain when completely cooked.
- Add pasta to the hamburger mixture.
- Sprinkle cheese on top.

tender), and put a dab of butter or sour cream, slivers of ham, and some spices in the middle. Then roll the chicken breast around the goodies in the middle so you have a "ball." Roll that in any gluten-free mix you have in the house (it really doesn't matter if it's a bread mix, pancake, or even muffin mix), or crushed potato chips. Then bake or deep fry, depending upon whether it's "diet day" or not, and you have a great meal that's probably too gourmet for your kids anyway.

Think ahead. If you're making bread, make an extra batch of dough and put it in the fridge or freezer. Then, someday when the rest of the family is having bread or rolls with dinner, pull out a handful of dough and roll it into a long "snake" or stick, or drop a few spoonfuls into muffin tins. You may want to drizzle a little butter on top for an added treat. Then pop them in the oven, and make fresh-baked bread sticks or biscuits. The house will smell great, and you'll feel like Mom of the Year!

So go ahead . . . live "la vida loca"—get wild, crazy, and *creative*!

Substitution Ideas

If a recipe calls for . . .

- soy sauce: use gluten-free soy sauce (at least a couple of national brands can be found at most major grocery stores) or Bragg's Amino Acids (similar to soy sauce).
- thickening with flour: use corn starch, arrowroot flour, or a bread mix (or any other mix) you have handy.
- coating with flour or bread crumbs (to fry or sauté): coat with a gluten-free bread mix, cornmeal, or crushed potato chips.
- croutons: cut some gluten-free bread into cubes, and deep fry or even pan fry in butter.

- pie crust: crush up old gluten-free cookies or cereal, mix with melted butter, and press into a pie tin.
- pasta: use gluten-free pasta (often the sauce on top is gluten-free anyway).
- flour tortillas: use corn tortillas, or use rice wraps found in Asian markets or the Asian food section of grocery stores.
- pasta pieces (as in rice pilaf, for instance): use crumbled pieces of gluten-free pasta.
- crackers: use rice crackers or Savory Thins.
- bun (for hamburgers or sandwiches): use gluten-free bread, corn tortilla, or lettuce wrap.
- sauce: try salsa, melted cheese, or mayonnaise mixed with ketchup.
- thickener for sweets: use dry pudding mix (several gluten-free varieties are available in the stores), or corn starch and sugar.

Quick Meal Ideas

Okay, you're ready to cook, or at least to prepare some quick treats! Here are some menu-planning ideas to get you going. Note that I refer to a number of products that can be gluten-free or not (e.g., peanut butter, jelly, cream cheese, etc.). Make sure that you check the status of each of these ingredients.

Breakfast
- Eggs, cooked any way your child will eat
- Egg in a basket
  - Butter both sides of a piece of gluten-free bread. Tear a hole in it, fry it in a frying pan, and drop an egg in the hole. Flip when the cooked side is golden brown. Cook until the other side is golden brown, too.
- Fruit
  - It's fun to dig out a scoop of kiwi or cantaloupe and put a spoonful of yogurt in it.
- Toast (gluten-free)
  - Remember, the breadmaker and slicer are lifesavers!
- Cereal
  - There are several commercial brands available at any grocery store. They're generally made with rice or corn, and do not have malt flavoring in them. Health food stores carry several gluten-free brands.
- Quesadillas (a warm tortilla with melted cheese inside)—Use corn tortillas, of course.

- Bacon
  - There are several gluten-free brands available at any grocery store.
- Sausage
  - There are several gluten-free brands available at any grocery store.
- Yogurt
- Smoothie
  - Fruit blended in blender with orange juice, milk, or ice cream. I usually try to dump some protein powder in there when the kids aren't looking.
- Instant breakfast
  - There are commercial brands that are gluten-free; you should check status.
- Grits or rice cereal, served with butter, cinnamon-sugar, or syrup on top
- French toast (made from slices of gluten-free bread)
- Pancakes
  - There are several excellent gluten-free pancake mixes available by mail (see Resource Guide at the end of this book for listings). Many health food stores sell gluten-free pancake/ waffle mixes.
- Waffles
  - There are several good mixes, and some excellent pre-made freezer waffles that you just warm in a toaster or toaster oven. The freezer waffles can be found in health food stores, or even in national grocery chains in the health food section.

Lunch

- Sandwiches (made with gluten-free bread)
  - Peanut butter and jelly, cucumber and cream cheese, ham, cheese—the only thing limiting your options (besides gluten) is your creativity!
- Waffle Sandwich
  - If you don't have any gluten-free bread handy, use a frozen waffle (toast it first) instead.
- Tamales or taquitos
  - There are several commercial brands sold at grocery stores.
- Quesadillas
  - Corn tortilla, of course.
- Fruit

- Hot dogs (gluten-free) (no bun)
  - There are several commercial gluten-free brands sold in grocery stores.
  - For a bun, try wrapping a corn tortilla around the hot dog, then heating in a microwave. The juices from the hot dog will steam the tortilla.
- Hamburger (no bun)
- Nachos
  - Corn tortilla chips with cheese melted on them. Feel free to add chicken, beef, veggies, beans, or any other leftovers you have.
- Tuna and mayonnaise on gluten-free toast or GF crackers
- Tuna melt
- Grilled cheese sandwich
- Grilled chicken on a bun or with lettuce wrap
- Macaroni and cheese
  - You can either buy gluten-free pasta and melt your own cheese on it, or health food stores now carry gluten-free varieties of "macaroni and cheese" in a box, much like Kraft or other commercial brands.
- Pizza
  - You can either make your own crust from a cookbook recipe or mix, or put pizza "fixin's" on a corn tortilla or piece of gluten-free bread.
  - There are several online and mail-order companies that sell excellent pre-made pizza crusts; stock up and freeze them.
- Spaghetti (Let your kids make the meatballs)
- Cheese and GF crackers
- Hard-boiled eggs
- Baked beans (check the brand) and gluten-free weenies or bacon
- Soup (travels well in a lunchbox in a small Thermos)

Dinner
- Hamburger
- Meatloaf
  - Put bread crumbs or crushed non-sweetened gluten-free cereal in if you have some available; otherwise do without and mix an egg, barbecue sauce, and the meat, then bake).
- Taco salad
  - Put tortilla chips on the bottom (they're the best part), salad, chicken or hamburger with taco spice, beans, grated cheese, and anything else you can think of. Top it with your favorite salad dressing.

- Spaghetti or other pasta (gluten-free)
  - Several commercial brands of spaghetti sauce are gluten-free.
  - Make meatballs (no breading, of course) to go on top.
- Macaroni and cheese
- Creamed tuna on toast
  - Mix tuna, cream, a dab of butter, and a teaspoon of corn starch to thicken it; then serve over gluten-free toast
- Tamales
- Taquitos
- Quesadillas
- Tacos
  - Most hard shells at the store are gluten-free. You may also use corn tortillas raw or deep fried in oil.
- Barbecued or steamed vegetables
- Soup
  - You can get very creative making soups. Use a gluten-free chicken broth for the base, or one of the several gluten-free brands of bouillon.
- Fish, shrimp, or any other favorite from the sea (no breading, but marinated in a gluten-free sauce and grilled or broiled is delicious!)
- Pizza
  - We make a few crusts at a time and freeze them, so that we can pull them out and put sauce, cheese, pepperoni, and anything else we want on them for a quick pizza.
  - Another quick option is to use gluten-free bread or a corn tortilla as the "crust," and add the toppings.
- Hot dogs (gluten-free)
- Shish kebobs

Explore New Cuisines

Keep your eyes open for gluten-free foods you may not have tried before. Recently we were eating at a Thai restaurant, and noticed many "rice wrap" dishes. Some of the wraps were cold and uncooked; others were deep fried to a crispy crunch. We asked to see the package for the rice wrappers, and were delighted to discover that they were 100 percent rice flour, and apparently gluten-free. We jotted down the name of the manufacturer and distribution company, called to confirm their gluten-free status, and asked where they distributed these wrappers in our area. Within minutes, we had the names of several Asian markets and grocery stores in our area that carried them.

- Tuna melt
- Chinese chicken salad
  - Use tortilla chips, rice crackers, or maifun rice (from Asian market) for crunchies.
- Teriyaki chicken
  - Most grocery stores carry gluten-free teriyaki, although it can be difficult to find at first.
- Polska Kielbasa
  - There are gluten-free brands in the grocery stores.
- Steak or other favorite meat
- Cabbage rolls
  - Inside the roll you can put hamburger meat, vegetables, rice, or any combination thereof.
- Chili
- Chicken nuggets (or you can use fish and make fish sticks)
  - Cut the chicken or fish into nuggets or sticks. Coat with anything you have handy: a bread or pancake mix, or barbecued potato chips. Fry in oil or bake.
- "Wraps"
  - Use corn tortillas to wrap just about anything. Salad with salad dressing, beans and rice, avocado and turkey . . . get creative!
  - Use rice wrappers, found in Asian markets, or even the Asian foods section of your grocery store. They can be used cold, as a soft wrap, or deep fried into a crunchy wrap like on a spring roll.

Side Dishes

- Rice
  - Don't be afraid to jazz it up. There are several pre-packaged Spanish rices (and other flavors) available at the store, or you can make your own. You can also put coconut milk in it to make it creamy.
- Potatoes
  - Cut new potatoes into small pieces and fry them in whatever seasonings you have available, bake your own french fries, or make mashed potatoes sometime other than Thanksgiving or Christmas.
  - Some brands of boxed "potato buds" are gluten-free.
  - Make twice-baked potatoes. (Cut open baked potatoes, mix "insides" with margarine, cheese; put back in and bake with cheese on top)
  - Potato salad

- Croutons for salad or soup
  - Either use the gluten-free bread you have to make these (cut in cubes, deep fry, roll in parmesan cheese or seasonings), or use tortilla chips as croutons.
- Refried beans
- Salad
- Vegetables, barbecued or almost any way you like them
- Applesauce

Snacks

- Chips
  - There are *many* flavors of gluten-free chips available at grocery stores! See the next chapter for some specific brands.
- Fried string cheese (roll string cheese in any gluten-free flour you have available and fry it up).
- Taquitos, quesadillas, tacos, tamales (made with corn tortillas)
- Nachos
- Corn Nuts
- Raisins and other dried fruit
- "Chex" mix
  - There is a gluten-free cereal available at many grocery stores or health food markets that's just like Chex—make the mix as you would Chex mix.

"Our family is in the car a lot, and I have a hard time coming up with easy, healthy snacks that travel well.
—Theresa M.

- Popcorn
- Cheese cubes with toothpicks in them and rice crackers
- Fruit rolls
- Lettuce wrapped around ham, cheese, turkey, or roast beef
- Rice cakes (check with the manufacturer; not all are gluten-free)
- Hard-boiled eggs or deviled eggs
- Applesauce
- Apples dipped in caramel or peanut butter (if you're sending apples in a lunchbox, remember to pour lemon juice over the slices; that will keep them from turning brown)
- Individually packaged pudding
- Jello
- Yogurt
- Fruit cups (individually packaged cups are great for lunchboxes)
- Fruit snacks (like Farley's brand)
- High-protein bars (e.g., Tiger's Milk, GeniSoy)
- Nuts

- Marshmallows
- Trail mix
    - Combine peanuts, M&Ms, dried fruit, chocolate chips, and other trail mix items for a great "on-the-go" snack.
    - Beware of commercial trail mixes—they often roll their date pieces in oat flour.
- The occasional candy bar or other junk food treat (see the next chapter for information on safe junk food)

So, Your Kid's a Little Picky . . .

All children can be picky at times. But sometimes, kids with celiac disease can be particularly finicky because they have a negative association with food—when they eat certain foods, it makes them feel icky. Hang in there; this too will pass. But in the meantime, here are a few ideas that may help.

- Use fun and unusual eating utensils. There are many different types of entertaining straws, plates, cups, and utensils that will pique your child's interest in food. Make sure mealtime doesn't *always* turn into playtime, however, or you'll be scraping "Rocket Raisins" off the top of the fridge for weeks.

- Make the food look fun. Whether you cut the food into interesting shapes or letters, make faces on the sandwiches, or dye the food fun colors, the way your child's food *looks* is just as important to him as how it tastes. Shaping your kids' food into letters can be a fun way to practice reading and spelling, too.

- Ask your child to help plan the menu. Sometimes we forget to ask our kids what *they* want to eat. Oh sure, giving them the freedom to select their own menus all the time may result in a diet consisting solely of pizza and peanut butter, but you might be surprised at how reasonable they can be. By sitting down together and planning an entire week's menu in advance, you will have the opportunity to discuss proper nutrition, practicality, and how to make healthy food choices. Once your child has suggested a certain food, you may find she exaggerates the meal's virtues, simply because it was her idea. Let her think whatever she wants, as long as she eats her broccoli!

- Redundancy is okay. If your child wants to eat the same dinner every day of the week, that's okay! We tend to think that variety is important, and to some extent that's true. But really, as long as her diet has a healthy balance of protein, vitamins, and other essential nutrients, it truly doesn't matter at all if your child eats the same thing for dinner seven nights a week. Keep in mind that this pattern probably won't go on forever. Furthermore, you should be thankful. It makes deciding what to have for dinner so easy!

- K.I.S.S.: Keep It Simple, Supermom. I know, it's not very gratifying to boil up some gluten-free pasta and drop a dollop of butter on it. We sometimes get carried away making gourmet meals that look pretty and make the kitchen smell good, but we need to remember that kids like it simple. Especially the picky ones.

Don't make a big deal of it. As frustrating as it can be to have a picky eater, it could be that you've unknowingly entered into a battle of wills. And we *all* know who always wins *those* food battles between parent and child. Calmly explain that it's okay if she doesn't want to eat her dinner, but whatever you do, don't let her have a snack afterwards! She won't starve to death, and you can bet that you'll make a point that extends far beyond that meal.

Junk Food

It's Crucial!

13

"I know this may not be the most important concern in the world, but are there any good junk foods that we can feed our son?"
—*Brad L.*

For better or for worse, junk food is a way of life these days. Even products that are camouflaged with packaging that promotes nutritional value with terms such as "healthy," "nutritious," "high protein," and "100% fruit" are often laden with sugar (disguised as "sucrose"), preservatives, saturated fats, and chemicals galore. That's why it's called *junk*!

Of course I'm not condoning an all-chocolate-and-chips diet. It's important to ensure that our children eat adequate amounts of protein (no, not peanut butter), calcium (no, not ice cream), vitamins and minerals (no, not chewable cartoon characters), and fiber (no, not fruit roll-ups). (See Chapter Twenty-Three for in-depth information on nutrition.) But as a firm believer in "everything in moderation," I do think that there is a time and a place for junk food.

It's Emotionally Healthy

For children who already have a restricted diet that can be construed as "strange," I think the commercial junk food products play a crucial role in helping them feel "normal." That candy bar or bag of chips makes a very "loud," nonverbal statement on behalf of your child: I can eat these, just like you can! It's comforting to these kids to get a treat—but not just *any* treat—it's a commercial product that anyone can buy in any store. It's worth the sugar high you'll endure for the next two hours.

Of course, there's also the ease factor for us parents: the ability to go into a grocery store and snag a candy bar or bag of chips off the check-out stand to satisfy our kid's sudden craving or hunger pang—an act so unappreciated by most parents!

Let Go of the Guilt

I have friends who think oranges are a splurge because they're high in sugar and calories, and their version of "junk food" is dehydrated fruit with carob chips (a great treat, don't get me wrong). And I have to admit that as secure as my husband and I are about our parenting philosophies, I'm sometimes stricken by guilt and try to pretend the bag of chips I'm holding belongs to some lady in the park who was just passing by and asked me to watch them for her.

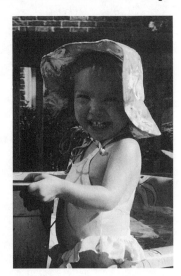

It *is* tempting to feel guilty about letting your child eat junk food, but remember the already-restricted diet he has, and let go of the guilt! You have more important things to worry about... like how you're going to explain to your zealously healthy friend how *his* child got a candy bar while you were watching him!

A Starter List

We generally do not list product names in this book. But because junk food can be crucial to the emotional well-being of your child, we have listed several products that, at the time of this publication, to the best of our knowledge, and with any other release-of-liability statements we can make, we believe to be safe for kids with celiac disease. Remember to check with the manufacturer to make sure the product's status is still gluten-free.

Chocolates/Candy Bars
- CADBURY

Cadbury Fundraising Bar	Dairy Milk	Mini Eggs
Cadbury's Bunnies	Easter Parade	Rum & Butter
Caramilk	Fruit & Nut	
Caramilk Roll	Golden Caramel	
Crunchie	Hazelnut	

- EATMORE
  Glosette peanuts   Glosette raisins

- EFFEM FOODS
  Snickers

- HERSHEY
  Almond Bar   Ovation Sticks: Coffee, Irish
  Almonds & Toffee   Cream, Mint, and Orange
  Almondillos   Petit Oh Henry
  Cherry Blossom   Pot of Gold:
  Giant Kiss   Assorted Mints
  Glossette Almonds   Cherries
  Glossette Peanuts   Chocolate-covered almonds
  Glossette Raisins   Excellence
  Golden Almond   Signature Pieces
  Hershey-ets   Solitaires
  Hershey's Chocolate Syrup   Special Dark
  Kisses   Reese:
  Jenny Lind   Crunchy Peanut Butter Cups
  Lowney Caravan   Miniatures
  Lowney Golden Caramels   Peanut Butter Cups
  Lowney Maraschino Cherries   Pieces
  Lowney Nut Milk   Skor
  Lowney Rosettes   Strand
  Oh Henry Bar   Truffles:
  Oh Henry Peanut Butter   With Dark Chocolate
                                    With Milk & Dark Chocolate
                                    With Milk Chocolate

- HERSHEY SEASONAL
  Advent Calendar   Pastel Kisses
  Caramel Egg   Pot of Gold Truffle
  Caramel Eggies   Reese Candy Cane
  Cream Eggs   Reese Minis
  Dinosaur Coin Bank   Reese Pastel Minis
  Easter Craft Eggies   Reese Peanut Butter Eggs
  Elf House   Reese Peanut Butter Trees
  Kisses   Reese's Pieces
  Kisses Cane   Solid Milk Chocolate Eggs
  Oh Henry Easter Eggs

- JUST BORN
  Marshmallow Peeps Eggs (Vanilla Creme Flavored Marshmallow Eggs)
  Mike & Ike Easter Treats (Cherry, Grape, Lemon, Lime and Tripleberry)
  Just Born Jelly Beans (Assorted Fruits, Berry, Spice, and Licorice)
  Peeps Jelly Beans (Marshmallow and Fruit Flavored Jelly Beans)

- NESTLE

Baby Ruth	Goobers
Butterfinger	RAisinets
Chunky	Nestle Treasures (**Except Crunch)
Nestle Milk Chocolate	Wonderball
Oh Henry!	SweeTARTS
Nestle Turtles	SPREE
Sno-Caps	Bit-O-Honey
Butterfinger BB's	Pearson Nips

- WONKA (Nestle) candies

Bottle Caps	Pixy Stix
Fun Dip	Runts
Gobstoppers	Tangy Taffy
Nerds	

- TOOTSIE ROLL INDUSTRIES

Tootsie Rolls	Dots Orange Cream Pops
Tootsie Pops	Crows
Flavor Roll	Tropical Dots
Twisties Caramel Apple Pops	Child's Play
Frooties Mutant Fruitant Pops	

- CHARMS COMPANY

Blow Pops	Charms Pops Family Fun
Charms Squares	Zip-A-Dee-Doo-Da Pops
Way-2-Sour Blow Pops	Pops Galore
Charms Sour Balls	

- CELLA'S CONFECTIONS
  Cella's Milk Chocolate Covered Cherries
  Cella's Dark Chocolate Covered Cherries

- CAMBRIDGE BRANDS

Junior Mints	Pom Poms Morsels

Sugar Daddy
Charleston Chew
Sugar Babies

Caramel-A-Lot
Candy Magic

Chips, Popcorn, and Nuts

- FRITO-LAY:
BAKED LAY'S brand Original Potato Crisps
BAKED LAY'S brand Sour Cream and Onion Potato Crisps
Baked TOSTITOS brand Original Flavor Baked White Corn Tortilla Chips
Baked TOSTITOS brand Unsalted Flavor White Corn Tortilla Chips
BAKEN-ETS brand Fried Pork Skins
CHEETOS brand Cheese Flavored Snacks (all varieties)
CHESTERS brand Butter Flavored Popcorn
CRACKER JACK brand Original
CRACKER JACK brand Original Fat Free
CRACKER JACK brand Butter Toffee
CRACKER JACK brand Butter Toffee Fat Free
DORITOS brand Cool Ranch Flavored Tortilla Chips
DORITOS brand Salsa Verde Flavored Tortilla Chips
DORITOS brand Taco Supreme Flavored Tortilla Chips
DORITOS brand Toasted Corn Tortilla Chips
DORITOS brand 3D'S brand Nacho Cheese Flavored Crispy Corn Snacks
DORITOS brand WOW! brand Nacho Cheesier Flavored Tortilla Chips
FRITO-LAY brand Bean Dip (all varieties)
FRITO-LAY brand NUT HARVEST Nuts (all varieties)
FRITOS brand Bar-B-Q Flavored Corn Chips
FRITOS brand Chili Cheese Flavored Corn Chips
FRITOS brand Corn Chips
FRITOS brand Dip Size Corn Chips
FRITOS brand Enchilada Cheddar Cheese Dip
FRITOS brand SCOOPS brand Corn Chips
FRITOS brand Sabrositas Lime 'N Chile Flavored Corn Chips
FRITOS brand Texas Grill Style Honey Barbecue Flavored Corn Chips
FRITOS brand WILD 'N MILD RANCH brand Flavor Corn Chips
LAY'S brand Potato Chips
LAY'S brand KC Masterpiece Potato Chips
LAY'S brand Salt and Vinegar Potato Chips
LAY'S brand Sour Cream and Onion Potato Chips
LAY'S brand Deli Style Potato Chips
LAY'S brand Deli Style Cheddar Potato Chips
LAY'S brand Deli Style Spicy Chili Potato Chips

LAY'S brand WOW! brand Original Potato Chips
MUNCHOS brand Potato Chips
RUFFLES brand Potato Chips
RUFFLES brand Cheddar and Sour Cream Potato Chips
RUFFLES brand KC Masterpiece Potato Chips
RUFFLES brand Reduced Fat Potato Chips
RUFFLES brand The Works Potato Chips
RUFFLES brand WOW! brand Original Potato Chips
RUSTLERS ROUNDUP brand Spicy Beef Stick
RUSTLERS ROUNDUP brand Beef Jerky
SANTITAS brand 100% White Corn Tortilla Chips
SANTITAS brand Restaurant Style Tortilla Strips
SANTITAS brand Restaurant Style Tortilla Chips
SMARTFOOD brand Reduced Fat White Cheddar Cheese Flavored
    Popcorn (Popped)
SMARTFOOD brand White Cheddar Cheese Flavored Popcorn (Popped)
SMARTFOOD brand Toffee Crunch Artificially Flavored Popcorn (Popped)
TOSTITOS brand 100% White Corn Bite Size Tortilla Chips
TOSTITOS brand 100% White Corn Tortilla Chips-Crispy Rounds
TOSTITOS brand 100% White Corn Restaurant Style Tortilla Chips
TOSTITOS brand Salsa-N-Cream Cheese Flavored Tortilla Chips
TOSTITOS brand Unsalted Flavor Baked White Corn Tortilla Chips
TOSTITOS brand Low Fat Salsa Con Queso
TOSTITOS brand Salsa Con Queso
TOSTITOS brand Salsa (Mild, Medium, Hot)
TOSTITOS brand Roasted Garlic Flavor Salsa
TOSTITOS brand Sweet and Zesty Salsa
TOSTITOS brand Ultimate Garden Flavor Salsa
WAVY-LAY'S brand Potato Chips
WAVY-LAY's brand Au Gratin Flavored Potato Chips

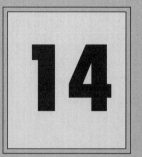

When You're Not There

Sitters, School, and Other Scary Situations

Letting Go

Letting your child out of your sight may be one of the most difficult steps you take. But it's important for your child and for you. If you're well prepared, and if you prepare the people around you, you will be at ease leaving your child at school, day care, church, camps, and in the care of babysitters, grandparents, friends, and other caretakers.

If you have truly given your child responsibility for her diet, depending upon her age and developmental stage, she should be able to make good food choices while you're away. Stress the importance of not cheating, and then give her a chance to prove herself.

Mistakes will be made, but everyone will learn from them. *Deal with it; don't dwell on it.*

Babysitters in Your Home

Having caretakers in your home should cause little or no concern to you if you've followed some of the guidelines outlined early on in this book.

- **Educate the caretaker.** Make sure the person watching your child has a good grasp of the diet and its importance. Give them a copy of the short explanation of celiac disease in the Appendix, or the book itself. Go over product information, focusing most on your child's favorite foods and likely temptations. Discuss menu and snack ideas, and provide lists of safe and forbidden ingredients. They need to know that if your child does accidentally get gluten, it's not an emergency. There is no need to panic, or to call 911 or a doctor. They don't need to call you immediately, but should let you know when you get home.

- **Leave pre-prepared food.** It's best if you can leave an entire meal, fully prepared, so there are no questions or mistakes. If you don't have time to prepare something in advance, leave a frozen entree that you know is okay.

- **Remember your notebook.** Remember that notebook you've put together? The one with all of the product information, manufacturers' correspondence, and general information on celiac disease? Leave it out where the babysitter can refer to it, if necessary.

- **Mark foods and plastic ware.** Hopefully, you have been marking all of your containers and products, as well as your plastic ware with leftovers, with a clear "gluten-free" designation. This will avoid any confusion when your child decides that it's time for an after-dinner snack.

- **Show the sitter the gluten-free treats drawer.** Instruct the sitter that your child's treats may come *only* from this area. Now is when having a separate drawer or cupboard will really pay off.

School

Anyone who has walked their child to her first day of kindergarten and spent the rest of the day crying in their car in the school parking lot knows it's hard enough to send the kids to school when they *don't* have dietary restrictions. But how do we send our children to school—where they'll be away from us for hours, day after day, snacking, eating lunch, swapping food items with friends, and enjoying birthday parties and holiday festivities—without our supervision?

With planning and preparation, it can be done. There *will* be mistakes, so brace yourself for the frustration. With a little extra effort on your part, though, the accidents will be minimal, and you can send your child to school with peace of mind.

- **Educate your teachers and principal.** Set a meeting with your child's teacher(s) and principal. The best time to do this is a day or two before school starts for the year. The teachers are usually at school setting up their classrooms, but they're not yet distracted with new students, parents, and classroom responsibilities. Provide the teachers, principal, and the school nurse, if you have one, with clear, concise written materials explaining celiac disease and your child's diet. Give them a short written summary of what your child can and can't eat (see page 211), and a copy of this book, if you feel it's useful. Make sure they understand the severity of accidental gluten ingestion. Remind them that they should contact you if there are any questions, rather than taking a chance.

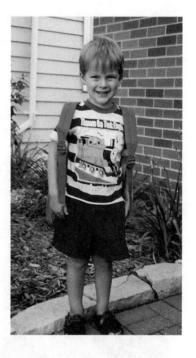

- **If any food is prepared by the school staff, use your judgment.** Most of the time, the people in charge of preparing food for children in a preschool or school setting are already used to dealing with lactose intolerance, peanut allergies, and other dietary restrictions. Talk to the dietitian or person in charge of food preparation. Go over the menu plans, discuss the foods your child can and can't have, and talk about the importance of using clean utensils to avoid cross-contamination. If you feel comfortable with the person's understanding and acceptance of the diet, give them the opportunity to accommodate your child's special diet. You always have the option of sending in your own meals if you think it's not working out.

- **Give the teacher a stash of gluten-free treats.** A large bag of Halloween-sized individually wrapped candies works well, and because they're individually wrapped, the teacher can keep them in a cupboard without the threat of ant invasions. Let the teacher know that these treats are to be used *any* time there is a special event during which treats will be served. Make sure the treats are your child's favorite; you don't want her feeling like she's being short-changed. If your child has a good grasp of her diet, let the teacher know that she can decide whether or not to dip into the treat stash.

- **Get a schedule of classmates' birthdays.** Teachers are glad to provide you with a listing of everyone's birthdays. This way you know in advance when there will be parties. You can coordinate with the other child's parent, or send your child in with her own cupcake or treat. If there's a surprise event, your child always has the stash of candy you've given the teacher.

- **Find out ahead of time about holiday parties.** Check the teacher's schedule to get dates for classroom parties, such as Halloween and Valentine's Day. Put the dates on your calendar as early as you can, so that you can prepare special party food to send in with your child.

- **It's best *not* to risk celebrating your child's birthday with gluten-free cupcakes.** It's possible that everyone in your child's class

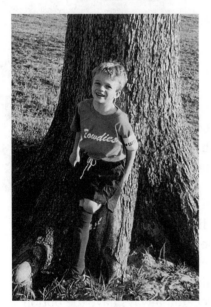

might like your homemade gluten-free cupcakes. On the other hand, there may be one kid who, for whatever reason, takes one bite and spits it across the classroom, declaring, "What IS this stuff?" You can bet your child won't forget that incident for a very long time. It's best not to risk it.

Instead, bring in ice cream bars or ice cream sundaes. Or, if you can't do frozen foods, bring cutely decorated candy bars or goodie bags filled with candy (brands that everyone knows). It will bring your child immense pleasure to share treats with the class that she can eat too (and kids like that stuff better than cupcakes anyway!). Of course, you will want to be sensitive to any of your child's classmates who might have peanut or other allergies, and choose treats that everyone in the class can enjoy.

- **Ask for liberal restroom privileges.** Many teachers restrict the number of times children are allowed to go to the restroom, or they ask children to wait until a more appropriate, less disruptive time. Let the teacher know that your child's condition may require a hasty trip to the restroom, and that she should under no circumstances be restricted from going. You may even want to establish a little "code" between your child and her teacher, so that she can inconspicuously dismiss herself. It's a little less embarrassing than having to ask.

- **Have your child bring a bag lunch.** This seems so obvious, and yet parents who contact R.O.C.K., our support group, agonize over how to feed their kids at school. Some, if not most kids bring their lunch to school anyway, so it should really be a non-issue.

- **Try to find a way your child can buy lunch one or more days per week.** While taking a lunch does seem such a common-sense solution to the school lunch issue, it is really nice if there is any way to have your child buy lunch once a week or so. Not for your convenience, of course, but for the feeling of "fitting in" that your child will experience. While every school is different, most lunch providers are contracted by the school. Try to work through your principal to get in touch with the lunch provider and determine whether there are any meals—or even any portions of meals—that your child can eat. It can be done! Our son buys twice a week. Yes, it takes a lot of time on our part, and a lot of cooperation from the lunch provider. And no, on those two days, he can't eat everything they serve. But even if he can eat a side dish, it's important to him, and that makes it important to us.

- **Talk to the adult lunchtime supervisors.** Kids will swap food. It's an age-old tradition, and it's not likely to stop with your child. Aside from the likelihood of getting gluten, your child may end up hungry. Sometimes your child's goodies are "better" than the other child's, and it makes your child so proud that she'll gladly give them all away, to be left with nothing. So the best you can do is explain to your child why she can't trade food with her buddies, and make sure the lunch area monitors are keeping an eye out for swappers. (If your child receives special education services, food swapping is something that can be addressed in a behavior management plan, if it is a significant problem. See Chapter Twenty-Five.)

- **Learn about federal laws that may cover your child.** There are several federal laws that apply to children with celiac disease at school (particularly if they are receiving special education). See Chapter Twenty-Five for information that may be relevant to your child.

Home-schooling

Some parents choose to home-school in order to avoid the perceived hassles of sending their children with celiac disease away to school. While home-schooling can be an excellent option for educating children, the decision should be made for personal and educational reasons, *not* because of a child's restricted diet. Generally, parents can overcome any obstacles they imagined would prevent their child from attending school by packing a lunch for their child or by working with the school to make sure it is safe for her to buy lunch.

Class Presentations on Celiac Disease

Depending upon your child's age, you may want to consider giving a presentation to her class. This is only a good idea if your child buys into it. If she's reluctant, don't push it—you're likely to thoroughly embarrass her. Most kids beyond third grade would rather not tell "the world" about their celiac disease, but for younger kids, a class presentation, ideally given early in the school year, can accomplish many things.

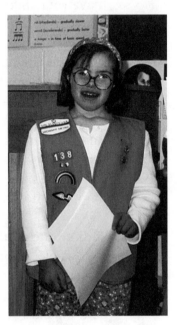

Most importantly, you will be educating the child's teacher and friends. Chances are, they already realized that your child "couldn't eat some things," and they may have even been a little fearful or concerned. A class presentation will make everyone feel more comfortable, and with any luck, it will minimize the likelihood that kids will offer their food to share, or will make fun of your child.

Here are some points to emphasize:
- This is a relatively common condition, and a lot of people have it and don't even know it.
- Your child is perfectly healthy as long as she stays on a gluten-free diet.
- This is no different from kids who have an allergy to peanuts or chocolate or some other dietary restriction.
- It's not contagious.

Not only are you filling people in on your child's condition, but you are educating twenty to thirty kids about celiac disease. And additional awareness of the disease is direly needed. Hopefully, your child's classmates will go home and talk to their parents about it, and the awareness will spread.

Teasing and Bullying

Whoever said, "Sticks and stones may break my bones, but words will never hurt me" had probably forgotten what it's like to be a child. Because words *do* hurt. And sadly, kids can be terribly cruel to one another. Even comments that are meant to be "playful" or are disguised as a joke can cause heartache.

Like a divining rod seeks out water, teasers and bullies seek out people who are the least bit "different"—like your child with celiac disease. Whether your child is being teased because of her diet, or because she has speech delays, needs to go to the nurse's office for medication, or has some other noticeable difference, there are several things you can do.

Most importantly, talk with your child about the situation. Find out exactly what the kid or kids are saying, and address that issue specifically. Our daughter used to whine, "Tyler called me dumb." Our response was, "Are you dumb?" She'd quickly say, "No, I'm really smart!" "Okay then, why does it bother you when he calls you dumb? Would it bother you if he called you a blue bug? No, of course not—because you're NOT a blue bug."

It's a little trickier when they're being teased about their diet, because they *do* have a special diet. But so what? Find out exactly what the kids are saying, and coach your child with some pat answers. If kids are saying, "You eat strange foods," your child can respond, "Well, they're not strange. They may be different from foods you eat, but they're good."

> "Sometimes I don't even want to go to school because some of the kids make fun of me because of my diet. I know they're just being mean, and my mom says to ignore them. But it's so hard, and it hurts so much."
> —Molly M., age 12

Most importantly, always remind your child what makes a good friend. A good friend doesn't dump you in favor of other friends; a good friend supports you when others are making fun; and a good friend never mocks or says mean things. Pick out some of your child's friends who are true friends, and use them for examples. Make sure that they know how important it is to always *be* that good friend, too.

If helping your child come up with snappy comebacks and lectures on friendship aren't working, talk with the bullying child yourself. If that doesn't work, go to the parents and teachers.

If all else fails, your child may need some formal counseling to deal with the teasing. Teasing is *not* to be brushed off as petty or unimportant. It can be devastatingly hurtful, and needs to be dealt with.

Crafts

Not only should your child not *eat* gluten, but if she is very young, it's usually a good idea for her to avoid *playing* with gluten, also. This is *not* because gluten can be absorbed through the skin. In fact, it cannot (see page 55. But if you remember back to your early days, you know it's just about impossible to resist taste-testing the Play Doh or the salt-and-flour dough that was molded into shapes and then hardened. Play Doh is made with flour, and is therefore, of course, laden with gluten. Even if your child isn't a nibbler, there is the chance that some of the Play Doh or paste will get stuck under her fingernails, and could be transferred to her mouth when she eats "real food."

You may make gluten-free play clay, paste, papier mache pulp, and other craft products and give them to your child's teacher to keep on hand (better yet, help in the class those days!). You can come up with your own recipes, but the following recipes will get you started*.

Play Clay**
1 one-pound box of baking soda
1 cup corn starch
1¼ cups cold water

Stir together baking soda and cornstarch in saucepan. Add water and cook over medium heat until mixture reaches consistency of moist mashed potatoes (approximately 10-15 minutes.) Remove and put on plate. Cover with a damp cloth. When cool enough to handle, pat until smooth.

Another Version of Play Clay
½ cup rice flour
½ cup corn starch
½ cup salt
2 tsp cream of tartar
1 cup water
1 tsp cooking oil
food coloring

Mix ingredients together, then cook, stirring constantly, for three minutes, or until mixture forms a ball. This clay may be stored in a plastic zippered bag, and will keep for several weeks.

Papier Mache Pulp
Many papier mache recipes contain flour, glue, and resin. Your child probably won't be tempted to taste-test the pulp, but just in case, you should use a gluten-free recipe for your papier mache projects.

2 cups gluten-free flour (any mix will do)
2 tsp xanthan gum (available from any health food store)
1½ cup water
¼ cup white glue

---

* Most suggestions from Celiac Disease Listserv archives, St.JohnMaelstrom. See Resource Guide for instructions for accessing the Listserv.
** Recipe from Arm & Hammer Baking Soda.

Mix ingredients thoroughly, adding the flour, xanthan gum, and glue to the water a little at a time. Stir the mixture frequently with a wire coat hanger or whisk. The objective is to get a smooth, even mixture with no lumps or air bubbles. Tear newspaper into long, thin strips. Dip the paper into the pulp mixture above and scrape the excess off with your fingers. Layer the pulp-covered strips onto your project.

Paste
¾ cup gluten-free flour
½ tsp xanthan gum
2 cups cold water
2 cups boiling water
3 tbsp. sugar
1 tsp salt

Mix the flour and the cold water. Add that mixture to boiling water and allow it to return to a boil. Remove from heat and add the sugar and salt. Let the entire mix cool and thicken. Once the mixture cools, it is ready to use.

Edible Soy Nut or Peanut Butter Play Dough*
2 cups peanut butter or soy nut butter
1 cup honey
2½ cups powdered milk
1 cup powdered sugar
Use a strong mixer

Edible Play Dough *
⅓ cup margarine
½ tsp salt
⅓ cup light corn syrup
1 tsp gluten-free vanilla extract (or other flavoring)
1 lb. powdered sugar

Mix all ingredients except sugar together. Then add powdered sugar. Knead the mixture. Divide and add food coloring. Refrigerate to keep from spoiling.

Another Edible Peanut Butter Play Dough*
1 cup peanut butter
½ cup honey
1 – 1½ cups powdered milk

---

* Store all edible dough in the refrigerator. Discard after one week.

Spoon the peanut butter into a mixing bowl. Pour in the honey. Mix in 1 cup of powdered milk and blend until smooth. Add up to 1/2 cup more powdered milk if you want a thinner consistency.

Beeswax

Beeswax has many benefits as a modeling compound:
- Beeswax is very clean; it doesn't get stuck in the carpet, in clothing, or in hair.
- Its colors stay true.
- It doesn't need special containers, and doesn't dry out.
- You don't have to make it; it is available in small sheets at teaching supply or craft stores.
- It's easy to use. Just hold it in your hands for a few minutes to warm it up and make it pliable. To save something you've made, just let it get cold. That shape can then be modified just by warming it again in your hands.

Cooking Projects

Schools often have special cooking projects. Depending upon what the class is making and how well your child's teacher understands celiac disease, it may be okay to let your child cook or decorate food products.

But if the flour will be furiously flying, or if you're worried that your child may nibble along the way, there are fun options. One mother who didn't want her child cooking with gluten-containing ingredients had the teacher assign her son to be the class photographer during a cooking project, so that he could be involved, yet was not dealing directly with the food products.

Maintain close communications with your child's teachers to determine the best way to handle the situation. Maybe you can come up with a gluten-free menu, or at the very least, ask the teacher to keep a close eye on your child.

Team Sports' Snack Time and Pizza Parties

If your child participates in team sports, she will have to learn to deal with the team snack frequently handed out to each child after each game. Generally, each family will assume snack responsibility, rotating through the roster. That means a dozen or so families may be bringing snacks to the game. Don't expect them to provide gluten-free snacks for your child, and don't be offended when they bring cookies or cupcakes that your child can't have. Just make sure you have brought a snack for your child (or better yet, that she has brought her own!), and politely refuse the cupcake. If you feel it's appropriate to explain, go ahead.

You may be pleasantly surprised to find that some parents will call you before their snack day and ask what a good gluten-free snack for the entire team might be. But don't expect that. To get agitated because other parents are not concerned about your child's diet is just going to create an additional stress in your life that you don't need.

After games, especially victories, it seems everyone shouts, "Let's go out for burgers without the bun!" Well, okay, it's really pizza they're shouting for, but one can dream. So how to handle the pizza party victory celebrations? You can go to the games prepared with your child's gluten-free pizza in hand, or you can find something else on the menu that she can eat. Many pizza parlors are surrounded by other fast food joints, so you can run across the street and buy a burger without the bun, and return to the pizza parlor for a salad and victory celebration.

"My daughter plays softball, and after each game, a snack is handed out. I've told a few of the moms about Tally's diet, but they either forget or just don't care. Every snack turns out to be something she can't eat; it's really starting to make me mad that they're so inconsiderate."
—Stacie H.

Church and Holy Communion

If your church or synagogue serves cookies or other baked goods after the service, be sure to remember to bring a good gluten-free alternative for your child.

If your child attends a church in which she will be receiving communion, remember that the wafers are *not* gluten-free! Talk to your priest, minister, or pastor about how a gluten-free wafer may be hosted. Also be aware that if people have bread crumbs on their mouth when they receive the wine, there could be contamination. In the past, some priests have insisted that "the staff of life is wheat," and cannot, therefore, be substituted. But most priests are willing to work with you on a variety of gluten-free options. For instance, they might allow rice crackers or slices of toasted rice bread as substitutes for wafers.

You may want to try making your own wafers. Ask your priest if he knows about any particular requirements, and then give it a try.

Communion Substitute
6 cups gluten-free flour (or mixture)
1 cup olive oil
1 cup milk
2 eggs
Dash of xanthan gum

Mix together, knead, and roll so that it is very thin. Cut into sections. Bake at 350 degrees for 7-8 minutes on each side. Break into small pieces when cooled. May be frozen.

Camp-Outs and Away-Camps

Ah, s'mores by the campfire. But not for your child, right? Wrong! Most chocolate is gluten-free, and many commercial brands of marshmallows are, too. Your child *will* have to do without the graham cracker, but there are some good substitutions. Gluten-free cookies, for instance, are even *better* than graham crackers! So again, it's just a matter of being prepared and having the right attitude.

> "My son's Cub Scout pack is going on a three-day camp-out next month, and I'm really disappointed that he'll have to miss it. How do other parents deal with sending their celiac kids away to camp?"
> —Ray H.

You're not very likely sending your four-year-old away to camp, so chances are, your child is old enough to understand her diet and the importance of sticking to it. If a parent you know is going, designate him or her to help at meal times. But remember to give your child most, if not all, of the responsibility.

If it's an event that takes place annually or on a regular basis, talk to someone who has been before. If you don't know anyone who has been, talk in advance with the leaders or chaperones. Ask how meals are prepared, what the typical meals are, and whether the accommodations have a full kitchen. You may want to mention your child's special diet, and see where they fall on the scale of "getting it."

Coolers are Cool—Send Food!

If you have talked with the camp counselors about the food situation and it seems there will not be a reliable source of gluten-free food available through the camp, pack a cooler with enough safe food for the entire stay. It's really not as hard as it may sound at first, especially if you also pack a suitcase full of non-perishable goods.

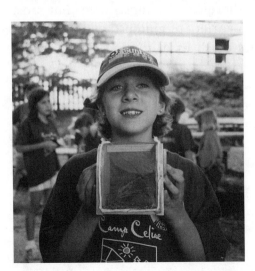

The suitcase of non-perishable items can contain cookies, crackers, bread, pancake mix, soups (the kind you just add water to, as well as pre-made canned soup), chili, and anything else your child will want. Most important items on the checklist: marshmallows and chocolate! Remember to mark every item with a big "GF," so there won't be any questions during your child's stay.

Pack a cooler full of eggs, cheese, fruit, milk (probably at the camp already), deli meats, Jell-O, pudding, hamburger meat, steak, chicken, or any other foods your child likes. If there are no cooking facilities (wow, they're *really* roughing it!), she can make do with the deli meats, cheeses, and pre-cooked foods. Don't forget to load the cooler with uncontaminated containers of "spreadables" such as

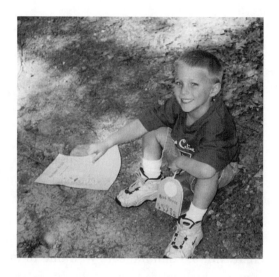

margarine and sour cream. It's also a good idea to throw in some salad dressing, ketchup, and mustard. Many of these things come in squeeze containers that are not only handy, but highly resistant to contamination. Once at the campsite, transfer the perishables to a refrigerator, if there is one. If there isn't one available, make sure there is plenty of ice to keep the food cold.

Who will prepare the food will depend upon your child's age and abilities, the length of stay, the type of food being cooked, and your good ol' parental judgment. If your child can prepare her own food, great. That's always best, because as we've stressed throughout this book, your child needs to learn to be responsible for her own diet.

Whether or not you should pack pots and pans depends upon the length of stay and the type of food that will be prepared. Usually camping food is prepared over a roaring fire on the end of a stick. It *is* a good idea to pack aluminum foil, which can be used as a "toaster" for a slice of gluten-free bread, or even a "frying pan" for sausage or bacon. It can also be used to coat a pot or pan that has been used to cook gluten-containing foods (it must still be washed before cooking gluten-free foods, even with a protective layer of foil).

If your child will be away at camp for an extended period and you're worried that the cooking facilities will be limited or coated with gluten, have your child bring a toaster oven to camp. Really, they're not that big, and assuming there is electricity at the camp, it can save you and your child some discomfort or annoyances.

Special Summer Camps

Some of the national support groups have kids' camps every summer. These are designed specially for children with celiac disease, and therefore accommodate the gluten-free diet without any questions or mistakes. See the Resource

Guide at the end of this book for information on organizations that sponsor special camps.

Should Your Child Wear a "Medical ID" Bracelet?

This is a personal matter that you will need to decide. There are pros and cons, but if you want my opinion (and I'm writing the book, so I get to give it!), the cons outweigh the pros.

The obvious pro is that people will know, especially in an emergency situation at a hospital or clinic, that your child must not ingest gluten. And if your child cannot communicate well due to an injury or underlying condition, emergency personnel can check the bracelet for her name, phone number, and any other identifying information engraved on the bracelet.

On the negative side, the sad reality is that most hospital personnel will not know what gluten is, much less whether or not a particular medication contains gluten. Furthermore, if it's a life-threatening or serious situation, you won't care if it does. There is even a chance that critical treatment of your child could be delayed while concerned hospital personnel try to figure out what gluten is, and whether or not it is a concern in the immediate treatment of your child.

These are the most serious concerns about this type of bracelet, but the other point to be made is one you will read throughout this book: Don't dwell on it. To wear a bracelet is a constant reminder to your child and everyone around her that she has "a condition." There is certainly no need for that, and the long-term psychological implications could be very negative.

Holidays, Birthdays, and Other Special Occasions

Holidays and special occasions—it seems as if they all revolve around food! These can be some of the most difficult times for our kids with celiac disease. They can feel left out, deprived, and even embarrassed. But with a little effort on your part, you can ensure that your child will be included and able to enjoy special occasions and the foods that usually go with them.

Rule number one: Don't expect others to accommodate your child's special diet. If they offer and you feel it's appropriate to take them up on their offer, go for it. But to expect them not only to remember that your child has a special diet, but then to understand how to accommodate it is being a bit presumptuous on your part.

Before heading out to a celebration for a special occasion where you know food will be

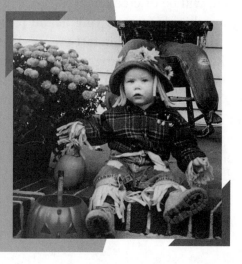

served, make sure your child has filled up at home. If you have a favorite fast-food chain where you can rely upon getting a gluten-free meal, have him eat on the way.

Try to find out in advance what will be served, both for the main course and for the dessert. Exactly how you do this will depend upon how big the party is and whether it will be held at a restaurant, catered, or hosted by a friend. It will also, of course, depend upon your relationship with the host. But in any 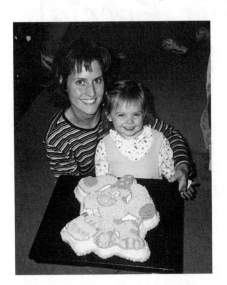 case, you'll want to make sure that it doesn't sound as though you're "hinting" that you'd like the host to prepare something special for your child. In fact, you can ask about the menu more as a matter of curiosity, without ever mentioning your child's specific dietary restrictions, or else you can be ambiguous and say, "Our family has some dietary considerations; do you mind telling me what you're planning to serve so that we can prepare?" If it's a good friend, you can, of course, be up front with your inquiries. The important thing to remember is that it's not the host's responsibility to accommodate your child's diet—it's yours.

Assuming the meal will not be gluten-free, bring a meal for your child that is as close to what they're serving as possible. For dessert, have him tell you what he'd like to have, and bring that, too. If your child will be attending the party without you, give the food to an adult in charge, and ask them to inconspicuously serve your child his special meal. Most adults are sensitive enough to be aware of the embarrassment your child could feel if they make a big deal about the different food you've provided, and will be discreet.

If you have stuffed your child before arriving at the party, or if you have provided a special meal, it's appropriate, and in fact even a good idea, to let your child take some of the food he *can* eat (assuming you know that some of the food being served is, in fact, gluten-free). However, if the plates are pre-served and there are gluten-containing portions, don't let him eat the gluten-free items unless you're certain that they have not been contaminated by the gluten-containing foods. Even if he's just going through the motions of eating the meal, he will feel included, and it is less likely that questions will come up that might attract unwanted attention to him.

Birthdays

Happy birthday to you,
Happy birthday to you.
There's gluten in cake,
And in many ice creams, too.

The center piece of so many birthday parties seems to be gluten. As a result, what should be a joyous celebration can turn your stomach into knots.

Relax. There is no reason that your child should miss the wonder of birthday parties—whether they're his own or someone else's. A little preparation will ensure your child will have a great time, regardless of the food served.

School parties can catch you off guard, because you're focusing on homework and class activities, not other kids' birthdays. Be aware that most kids have some sort of a celebration in school, so be sure to get a list of the birthdays of all the children in your child's class at the beginning of the school year. Mark them on your calendar right away, or you're sure to forget one, and you'll drown in guilt when your child gets home from school that day complaining that all the *other* kids got cupcakes. If one of the children's birthdays falls on a weekend, call the parent in advance to see if they plan to do the class celebration on Friday or Monday.

Going to parties shouldn't be a problem, either, even though these days it seems that "birthday party" is synonymous with pizza. That's okay, especially if you've perfected a pizza recipe for your child, or have found a good source of mail-order pre-prepared pizza. Bring your child's pizza, as well as a gluten-free cupcake or other special treat, and give it to the adult in charge. Make sure they understand how crucial it is that your child be given his special food, and ask them to be inconspicuous about giving it to him. Remember, too, that kids are there for the celebration and the fun, *not* for the food!

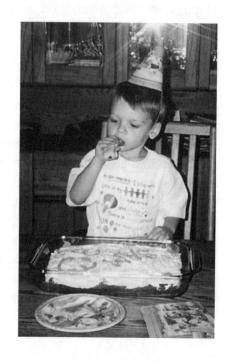

If the party is being held at a restaurant, bowling alley, or "fun zone," you can still find out in advance what will be served, and you can send a similar meal for your child. If the restaurant happens to serve hamburgers, salads, or other gluten-free meals, you may be able to arrange with the host parents for your child to get one of the gluten-free items on the menu.

If it's your own child's birthday party, plan to have hot dogs or hamburgers, or another gluten-free favorite. I don't recommend serving a gluten-free cake, even if you make the most awesome-to-die-for-gluten-free cake in the entire universe. Chances are, there will be one kid—probably the same kid who feels obliged to tell all the other kids at school that there isn't a tooth fairy—who will decide that he doesn't like the cake, and won't exactly be diplomatic in voicing his disapproval. You definitely don't want to cause your child the embarrassment he is likely to feel when that one child makes a scene.

So you may not want to take the chance. Serve frozen ice cream bars, or arrange in advance for individual hot fudge sundaes to be made by your local ice cream or frozen yogurt shop. The kids will love the change of pace!

Seasonal Holidays

Many candy manufacturers market seasonal items, and can verify that they are gluten-free. Do your homework in advance, and you will have lists of holiday candies that your child can eat. Stock up in advance, so that you're prepared to do the treat trade when your child brings home candy that he can't eat.

Christmas

It seems like every Christmas, elves appear from nowhere, handing out candy canes like they were, well, candy! Unfortunately, most come without a label, and are therefore no-nos.

Even if you find candy canes with ingredients listed and they appear to be gluten-free, teach your child to rinse the candy cane off before eating it. Washing it makes a gooey, sticky mess, but some candy canes are rolled in flour so that the plastic won't stick, and it's important to dissolve the outer layer of candy away, just in case.

There are several brands of candy canes that are verified to be gluten-free. Stock up on them and carry a few with you, so that when a well-meaning elf slips your child a candy cane, you'll be prepared to trade treats.

Here's the really good news: Little Timmy won't have to slip his piece of fruit cake into a napkin to feed to the dog under the table . . . he can just politely decline, reminding Aunt Betsy that hers *is* the most fabulous fruit cake in the world, but he can't eat it because it's loaded with gluten.

Easter

Once again, people with the best of intentions will be handing your child goodies laden with gluten. Be prepared with a well-stocked pantry so that you can do the treat trade. For better or for worse, every grocery store is loaded with commercial-brand candies, so that you can fill those Easter baskets with all sorts of safe treats. See Chapter Thirteen for some safe varieties.

Halloween

Take the time in September to find out which popular Halloween candies are safe. Chapter 13 lists many candies that were safe when this book went to print, but remember, just because something was safe last year doesn't mean it's okay this year. If your child is old enough, make sure he knows which candies he can and can't eat, because you can bet

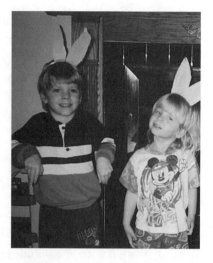

that he'll be itching to open his treats even before he's left the doorstep and yelled the obligatory thank-you over his shoulder. Make sure younger children understand that an adult needs to check the candy before they can eat it.

Keep a treat-trade basket at home, so that your child can make an "even" trade for the candies he gets that are not gluten-free. Then do what all parents do, and deplete his stash slowly enough that he doesn't notice, but quickly enough that the fights over candy before dinner can end and familial peace be restored.

And what about the traditional Halloween candied or caramel apples? Thankfully, many recipes for caramel coating and even the prepackaged coatings that you can buy at the grocery store are gluten-free. But you still need to check the labels and call the manufacturer. You may even want to volunteer to be the mom or dad who provides caramel apples for the Halloween party at school or your house of worship, so that you know for sure.

Passover

Passover is a blessed event, whether you're Jewish or not. That's because Passover is the only holiday that is celebrated almost entirely gluten-free!

Chametz (wheat, rye, barley, oats, and spelt) is forbidden during the Passover season, so foods marked "Kosher for Passover" are gluten-free, with one exception. Matzo (Matzah) is made with wheat and water, and is permitted. It is also ground into matzo flour and matzo meal, so avoid any product that contains matzo or "cake flour."*

Kosher products always have very clearly marked labels, so it's easy to identify all ingredients.

Thanksgiving

Without much extra effort, Thanksgiving can be celebrated with a wonderfully gluten-free feast. But you *do* need to pay attention, especially if you're eating at someone else's home.

---

* *Gluten-Free Living Magazine,* January/February 1999.

The stuffing, even though it is *inside* the bird, is a big no-no. No matter how careful you are, it *will* contaminate the turkey meat. The best idea is to stuff the bird with a gluten-free stuffing (see sidebar for suggestions on making gluten-free stuffing). If you would like to provide a traditional gluten-containing stuffing for your guests, prepare it separately and bake it in the oven. You can still pour turkey juices over it to end up with a wonderful "fresh turkey" flavor, but you won't have contaminated the entire bird.

Gluten-Free Stuffing

• Key Ingredient: Creativity

One of the coolest things about stuffing is that, just as there are no two snowflakes that are identical, there are no two stuffings that are exactly the same. Even if you follow a recipe, stuffing will vary every time you make it. So, if it turns out looking a little strange, it is your prerogative to declare, "That's the way *this* type of stuffing is supposed to look."

Our son loves rice (good thing, with this diet). So to make stuffing, I start with a rice base. What goes in at that point usually depends upon the leftovers we have in the fridge—old gluten-free bread, sausage, mushrooms, and of course the "usual" stuffing elements—celery, butter, and chicken broth (GF, of course). Get creative!

Most gravies are prepared with flour, and are obviously off-limits to your gluten-free child. But try substituting corn starch for flour, and your gravy will be just as good—maybe even a little lighter and better—than the traditional variety. You should always assume, when eating at other people's homes or at restaurants, that the gravy is prepared with flour, and should not be eaten by your child.

Some people worry about the turkey itself. You definitely *should* check to see if the bird has been injected or basted with any sort of sauce (soy or teriyaki, for instance). Most turkeys are just fine. Some people wonder if the food the turkey has eaten could contaminate the meat. They feel that to be safe they must buy a "free range" turkey (one that was raised in a natural, organic environment, usually without severe physical constraints). While this may be a choice based on health reasons, it is not an issue for people with celiac disease specifically, in my opinion.

Cranberries, sweet potatoes, green beans, Waldorf salad, and many of the other traditional Thanksgiving feast favorites can be made gluten-free, if they're not already. Okay, the rolls are off-limits, but are you going to be happy that the thorns have roses, or annoyed because the roses have thorns?

Restaurants
Can We Ever Eat Out Again?

"Our family used to enjoy going out to dinner at least one night a week. Now we can't do that anymore . . . or can we?"
—Susie A.

Whether you're going to a restaurant or a friend's house, eating out may not be as easy as it used to be, but it isn't impossible, either. In fact, it's much easier to go out and stay gluten-free than it is to go out and eat Kosher at a non-Kosher restaurant. Going out to eat is an important part of maintaining "normalcy" in your life. So dig out the good duds and work up an appetite, because it's time for a night out on the town!

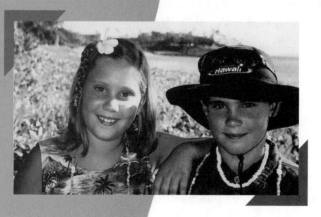

Rule number one before going out to dinner: Always have your child fill up before you leave. Even if you are going somewhere where you expect to have gluten-free menu items, it's nice to know her belly is full of safe food.

Restaurants

If you have a favorite restaurant, you can do your homework in advance, and feel comfortable going back and ordering safe items. Some large restaurant chains have actually put together a list of their gluten-free menu items (bless them).

According to Josef Lageder, Executive Chef for La Costa Resort and Spa in La Costa, California, many restaurants and resorts are well equipped to deal with special diets.

"Most chefs are prepared and willing to make accommodations for special dietary considerations," he says. "It's important to give us advance notice, up to a week or two if possible, and try to talk directly with the executive chef. Ask them to fax you a menu so that you may choose a meal, and talk with the chef about how to prepare it so that it is strictly gluten-free. In some cases, dedicated utensils can be purchased and used to ensure there is no cross-contamination."

He says that even if you are staying for a week or more, they are happy to accommodate the diet for every meal, if you have talked with them in advance.

But what if you don't have a chance to check out the restaurant in advance? There are some important tips to keep in mind.

- **Ask a lot of questions—don't be shy about it!** Why is it that when the waiter or waitress comes to the table to take our order, we feel like we are allotted twenty seconds to place an order? We feel that if we ask too many questions or make too many special requests, we're just a big pain in their necks. Well, that's fine. Be a pain. Ask lots of questions, even if your waiter seems annoyed. If you get the impression that your server isn't really "getting it," ask to talk with the chef or manager. Oftentimes, if you call the restaurant before the dinner rush (before about 3:00), you can talk directly with the manager or chef. You can even figure out what to order that evening, and save the hassle of dealing with the server.

- **Let your child order for herself.** She needs to get in the habit of asking for the burger "without the bun," and deal with the quizzical looks. Once she is able to decide what she wants (with your guidance, of course), let her place her own order.

- **Don't assume.** While it's true that many corn tortilla chips are gluten-free and not fried in the same oil as flour chips, don't order nachos for your child without checking to be sure. Confirm with your server that the hamburger is 100 percent beef (no fillers added), and that the burgers are not cooked on the same surface as the buns. Check to make sure the fries are not coated with anything, and the oil that they're cooked in is not used for other gluten-containing items such as onion rings or "chicken fingers."

- **Bring your own salad dressing.** Unless your child likes straight oil and vinegar, you shouldn't take a chance on the salad dressing. Most large restaurant chains do use commercial brands, so if it's a restaurant that you go to frequently, find out what kind of ranch dressing they buy (for instance), and then check with the manufacturer to make sure it's okay.

- **Consider bringing your own pasta.** Most chefs are glad to cook up a pot of pasta that you provide. Be sure to explain to them that they must use clean, dedicated utensils and water. Then ask them to top it with a little butter or pasta sauce, and you have a fresh pasta dinner. Generally you will not be asked to pay an additional charge for this (but be prepared to offer a generous tip!). It's a good idea to call the restaurant in advance if you plan to bring your own pasta.

- **Don't be afraid to ask for your child's meal to be prepared differently.** If the chicken sounds good, but it's breaded and fried, ask to have it grilled or broiled without the breading. People make special requests all the time.

- **Request a server.** If you eat at the same place often, you may find that the server remembers you and your special requests. If you're lucky enough to have such an astute waiter or waitress, request him or her and ask for "the regular."

- **Remember to bring a dessert for your child.** Unless you check, the ice cream and typical restaurant desserts can't be trusted. Since you don't want your child to feel left out, it's best to always go there prepared. In this case, you should probably bring something small but tasty such as a gluten-free candy bar, and there is generally no need to get approval from management in advance (some restaurants do have rules against bringing in your own food, but most are understanding when they understand the circumstances.)

- **Tip generously.** If the server, manager, or chef was accommodating, tell them you appreciate it by giving a generous tip.

- **Bring a "restaurant card."** You can either copy the sample on the next page, come up with your own, or purchase one from a support organization. (Several of the national groups listed in the Resource Guide at the back of this book have them.) The least expensive and easiest option is to make several copies; that way you won't have to ask for the card back. Present it to your server, make sure she understands it, and ask her to give it to the chef. Make sure they understand that if they have any questions, it's important that they ask you. You'll be pleasantly surprised how well received this approach generally is. Sometimes the chef will even come to your table to personally discuss the preparation methods.

RESTAURANT CARD

I have celiac disease, which means it is very important that I do not eat gluten. Gluten is in wheat (and wheat flour), oats, rye, and barley (malt). It can also be hidden in additives, spices, and condiments. Please make sure my meal does not contain any of the ingredients listed above, as well as the following additives:

- Hydrolyzed vegetable protein (HVP)
- Modified food starch (corn, rice, or soy are fine)
- (Customize your card to include any other forbidden ingredients that you do not care for or do not tolerate)

It's also important that my food doesn't touch other foods with gluten during the preparation process. Please don't cook my food in the same oil or use the same utensils you used for foods with gluten in them.
THANK YOU!

Generally Safe Bets

The following menu items are usually gluten free:
- Salad. Ask for oil and vinegar, or remember to bring your own dressing, and make sure they don't put croutons on the salad; explain to them that they can't just pluck them out. They can't ever go into the salad in the first place.
- Hamburger or cheeseburger, no bun. Explain to them that they can't just pick the burger out of a bun; tell them the bun must never touch the meat.
- Fries. Make sure they are not coated with anything, and that the oil used is not also used to deep fry gluten-containing items such as onion rings or "chicken fingers."
- Chicken, fish, or meats grilled or broiled without the usual breading or sauce.

- Nachos. Remember to check the chips and sour cream (modified food starch).
- Baked potato
- Fresh fruit platter
- Eggs (breakfast)
- Hash browns (if made from scratch)
- Fresh cheese slices (lunch)
- Cottage cheese

The Atkins Diet and Other Popular Low-Carb Diets

The Atkins diet asserts that a low-carbohydrate (*no* carbohydrates in the beginning), high-protein diet will result in weight loss. That means no bread, pasta, pizza, cookies, crackers, or other high-carbohydrate (and gluten-laden) foods.

I really don't know or care whether The Atkins Diet works for weight loss. But everyone dealing with a gluten-free diet should appreciate the road the diet has paved. Because of the huge popularity of the diet, people in restaurants are becoming accustomed to getting orders without the carbohydrates. No longer do order-takers at fast-food restaurants look at you as if you're from another planet when you ask for a burger without the bun! In fact, if you look around, there are lots of people tossing their buns aside or ordering their burgers without them. We can attribute this to either a huge rash of newly diagnosed celiacs, or The Atkins Diet (and similar popular low-carbohydrate diets).

Fast Food Restaurants

You may hate the idea of fast food restaurants, and you may hate the food itself. But the truth is that they're convenient, they're everywhere, and at many of them, you can find lots of gluten-free foods, some of which are even said to contain trace amounts of protein.

Of course, they probably don't have "burger without the bun" on their menu board, but the burger itself is likely to be 100% beef, so you can order it without the bun or even ask for a lettuce leaf to be wrapped around it in place of a bun. Some fries are coated to make them crispier, and they will not usually be gluten-free. But many of the fast food restaurants use only potatoes (and lots of salt) for their fries, and theirs are considered to be gluten-free.

Your safest bet is to contact the fast food restaurants that are closest to you, or that your child likes most. Most of the companies have representatives who

Contact information for Some of the Larger National Chains:

Boston Market
(800) 365-7000
www.boston-market.com

Burger King
(305) 378-7011
www.burgerking.com

Carl's Jr.
(800) 758-2275
www.carlsjr.com

Dairy Queen/Orange Julius
952 830-0200
www.dairyqueen.com

El Pollo Loco
(949) 399-2000
www.elpolloloco.com

In-N-Out Burgers
(800) 786-1000

Jack-in-the-Box
(800) 955-5225
www.jackinthebox.com

KFC (Kentucky Fried Chicken)
(800) 225-5532 (U.S.)
(800) 268-5435, ext. 1145 (Canada)
www.kfc.com

La Salsa/Green Burrito
(Santa Barbara Restaurant Group)
www.lasalsa.com

McDonald's
(800) 359-2904
www.mcdonalds.com

Popeyes Chicken and Biscuits
(800) 337-6739
www.popeyes.com

Subway
(800) 888-4848
www.subway.com

Taco Bell
(800) 822-6235
www.tacobell.com

Wendy's
(800) 82-WENDY
www.shc-wendys.com/gluten.htm

will be able to provide you with a complete list of their gluten-free menu items. If they don't have a list, ask specific questions about the beef patties, the fries, the milkshakes, and any other favorites that they serve.

You may want to ask if their fries or hash browns are deep-fried in dedicated oil. If they're not, and the fries are cooked with onion rings, turnovers, or other gluten-containing products, there is the likelihood of contamination. Whether or not the contamination from non-dedicated frying oil is enough to be of concern is a personal issue, and you should use your judgment on whether or not to allow your child to eat the product.

17 On the Road Again
Traveling Gluten-Free

There is absolutely no reason you should eliminate travel from your plans, just because of your child's dietary restraints. In fact, it's important for your child to gain the valuable experiences that travel will provide, and it's important for him to learn to travel on his own.

How you handle your travel plans will depend upon:

1. **Where you're going**
   - Will you be near major cities where they have grocery stores that carry items you know are gluten-free?
   - Is it likely there will be a health food store nearby?
   - Are you going to a foreign country where you won't have a clue what might be gluten-free, and where a language barrier might make things especially difficult?
   - Are there well-known chain restaurants nearby that you can call in advance to get a list of their gluten-free menu items?

2. **How long you'll be gone**
   • Will it be a short enough stay that you can bring your own food?
   • Will you be gone long enough to warrant bringing your own cooking appliances and utensils?

3. **Where you're staying (hotel, condominium, resort)**
   • Does it have a kitchenette or even a full-sized kitchen?
   • Is it a resort with an executive chef with whom you can discuss menu options?

4. **How you're traveling (cruise, driving, airlines, train)**

Regardless, there are some rules "of the road" that apply to any travel plans.

Do Your Homework Before You Go

In many cases, a little homework in advance will save you headaches (and tummy aches) on the road. If you're going to be staying in one area for an extended period, you may want to go to your local library, find the yellow pages for the closest major city, and look for a health food store that may carry gluten-free products. Call them in advance, and find out what gluten-free products they carry, if any. Often, if you tell them your favorite items and when you will be in town, they will order them for you. While you're looking at the yellow pages, you can also locate national chain restaurants that serve gluten-free items.

You might want to get in touch with one of the local branches of a national celiac disease support group (groups are listed in the Resource Guide at the

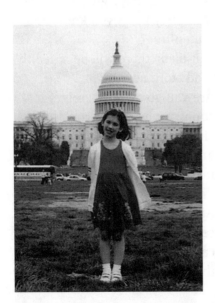

back of this book) to ask if they know of any good stores and restaurants in the area. Many of the groups are well-networked throughout the U.S. (and in other countries where the groups exist).

If you're going to a foreign country where you know nothing about the foods, you should study up before you go. Learn how to communicate "gluten-free" and "wheat-free" in the language of the country you will be visiting. If you know someone who speaks the language, you may want them to translate your child's restaurant card into the language of the country you'll be visiting before you go. (See page 110 for a sample restaurant card.)

Learn what types of spices and ingredients are generally used in the native cooking practices. For instance, in Mexico, corn is used much more widely than flour, and rarely are processed ingredients such as modified food starch added. In Japan, the soy sauce does not contain wheat; but in China, not only does the soy sauce contain wheat, but soy sauce is found in everything. Learn what you can about native cooking techniques by studying in the library or conferring with a local cooking school or executive chef of an international-style restaurant.

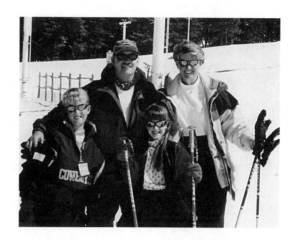

Kitchen in a Suitcase

Sometimes when my family travels, we bring an entire kitchen in a suitcase: toaster oven, mixes, pre-made and pre-sliced bread, gluten-free pastas, and cereal.

If you're going to be somewhere where you won't have access to grocery stores, you can bring canned goods (stews, chili, beans, tuna, and other "main courses") and boxed items that you would normally buy in a grocery store.

Most of the time, though, you're near a store and can stock up on all of your favorite snacks and meal items there. Don't forget to buy or bring plastic sandwich bags and small lunch bags, so that you can make a snack and take it on the run. It's also a good idea to buy aluminum foil, so that you can safely cook in ovens (don't ever set gluten-free food directly on the oven racks) or you can line baking pans that undoubtedly have been used for gluten-containing foods in the past.

Get a Room with a Kitchen or Kitchenette

It's always less expensive to prepare your own meals than it is to eat at nearby restaurants or at the hotel. Even many hotel rooms come equipped with a small bar area that can be turned into a kitchen, if necessary.

If the kitchenette has an oven, you don't even need to bring your toaster oven from home. Use the oven instead. Just put some aluminum foil down, put the oven on broil, and you have an extra large toaster oven.

With the gluten-free items you brought from home, and after a quick trip to the local grocery store, you're set to make toast, cereal, sandwiches, hot dogs, quesadillas, pasta, salad, and microwave popcorn. If you remember to bring cookie or cake mix (don't forget the cake pan, because most kitchenettes don't have them), you can even bake special treats. Don't forget the plastic utensils and plates, bowls, and cups.

Resorts, Cruises, and Hotel Restaurants

Because they cater to people who are spending huge amounts of money on their vacations, resorts and cruises are especially amenable to serving people on special diets. Most people just don't think to ask!

Call at least one month in advance, and talk with the executive chef. Let him know the age of your child, and send him your list of safe and forbidden products. Have him send you a menu that is age-appropriate, and then arrange a time

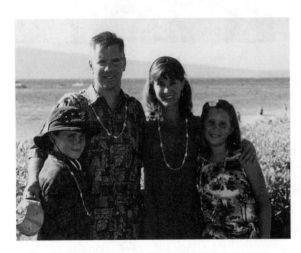

to call back and discuss the entire week's (or two-week) menu. Remind him that clean, dedicated utensils must be used in food preparation, and that cross-contamination is to be avoided. You'll be pleasantly surprised at how accommodating they will be!

If you haven't called in advance, you can eat at the hotel restaurant just as you would at any other restaurant. Either bring your own pasta and ask them to cook it with clean water and utensils, or review the menu and cooking process with the chef before you arrive, and decide upon a good gluten-free option.

For more information, refer to the previous chapter on eating out at restaurants.

Airline Food

In the olden days, the best you could hope for in airline food was a sandwich that your dog wouldn't have eaten, accompanied by a wilted salad and a piece of fruitcake. Today, unless you're on one of the econo-flights in which peanuts and sodas are the only meal you'll see for hours, the food is really very good.

Best of all, if you give most airlines a minimum of twenty-four hours' notice, you can request a gluten-free meal. In most cases, not only will it be gluten-free, but it will be good! But beware . . . the last time we were served a gluten-free meal, it came with a bagel—and no, it was not gluten-free. If you forgot to call in advance, all hope is not necessarily lost. You might get lucky enough to find that some of the snacks or meals being served to other travelers happen to be gluten-free. One mom told me recently about an experience in which she had forgotten to call in advance, but the flight attendants went into first class and found grilled chicken, mashed potatoes, salad, and several pieces of fruit.

As always, your safest bet is to bring a bag full of gluten-free treats that travel well, fill your child up with safe food before getting on the airplane, and check carefully before trusting that the gluten-free meal you've been given is truly gluten-free.

Hit the Road, Jack . . .

No matter where you're going or how you're getting there, you most definitely do not need to stay home because of your child's dietary limitations. In fact, you will most likely find that traveling is not that difficult at all. More importantly, it's a great experience for your child, and for the family as a whole. Think about *why* you're traveling, and focus on the joys of learning about new people, new places, new cultures, and the wonderful change of pace. Remember to keep it in perspective.

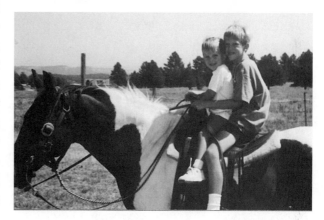

18

Cheater, Cheater, Gluten-Eater!
Intentional and Accidental Ingestion

One of the more difficult aspects of having children with celiac disease is that every time they're sick, we wonder whether it's because they've gotten gluten. We begin to question whether we inadvertently gave them something with gluten in it, and we start calling the manufacturers. Again. We wonder if maybe our kids weren't diligent in checking labels, or, worse yet, if they may have intentionally eaten something with gluten in it. And then again, we wonder whether they could be sick with something that's going around, and whether or not we should call the doctor.

What to Do When Your Child Gets Gluten

First of all, don't panic. Don't call 911 or the doctor. It is not an emergency. (If your child ingests massive amounts of gluten at one time—such as an entire pizza or loaf of

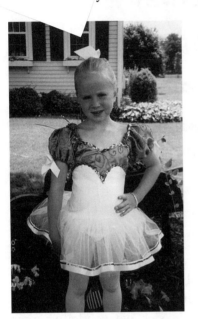

...ere is the possibility that her body could go into shock, in which ...ost definitely, be an emergency.)

...ortant that people, especially babysitters and teachers who may be ...your child when you're not around, understand that it is not like a peanut allergy or other condition in which a small portion of the "bad" food can cause an anaphylactic response. Eating gluten will not cause a threat to life, and does not require immediate medical attention.

Be prepared, though, because depending upon how much your child ate, how sensitive she is to gluten, and how much gluten was in the food, she *will* be uncomfortable. Usually children with celiac disease experience cramping, diarrhea, nausea, headache, fatigue, or some combination thereof. Some children vomit. School-aged children may have a little bit of trouble concentrating, and may do poorly on class assignments or tests. The symptoms generally appear within several hours or a day or two, and can last anywhere from a few hours to several days.

There aren't any over-the-counter medications that are very effective in treating the discomfort that celiacs feel when they eat gluten. Some people say that Pepto-Bismol™ helps; others say they get some relief from Maalox™; and still others recommend Alka Seltzer™, Immodium™, or garlic. But time is the only real healer, so get used to just waiting it out.

The bottom line is that accidents will happen, and so will intentional cheating. If your child has a clear understanding of the damage gluten does, and if she gets a severe reaction to gluten, she'll be less likely to experiment.

The Five Categories of Cheaters

Occasionally, a child will continually "make mistakes" or intentionally cheat. It's helpful to understand why a child cheats in the first place.

1. Doesn't Feel Any Symptoms

The kids who don't suffer any reaction when they eat gluten are notorious cheaters. And why not? They don't feel anything. Trying to tell them not to cheat on the gluten-free diet is as hard as trying to convince a teenager to stay out of the sun because it will cause her to have wrinkles or skin cancer when she's forty. Yeah, so what? I'm not forty now, and I won't be for *eons*, so what's the big deal?

While most celiacs suffer greatly when even trace amounts of gluten are ingested, it is not uncommon for children with celiac disease to be asymptomatic (feel no symptoms when they eat gluten) or suffer only mildly. As Chapter Twenty explains, teens entering puberty often go through a "honeymoon phase" in which they feel no effects whatsoever from gluten.

If your child doesn't experience the physical discomfort, you miss out on the wonderful power of aversion therapy. It's tough to break the cheating habit for kids who don't feel bad when they eat gluten, but there are some suggestions for dealing with your little cheater in the latter part of this chapter.

2. In Denial: Has Something to Prove

Anyone can go through denial, believing that the diagnosis of celiac disease was incorrect. People who feel no symptoms are extremely likely to experience denial, but so do people who suffer a great deal from symptoms. They may subconsciously "choose" to believe that they have something other than celiac disease—something, for instance, that is out of their control or does not require a dietary change. They may believe their symptoms are attributed to irritable bowel syndrome (IBS), stress, or lactose intolerance.

In an effort (usually subconscious) to "prove" to themselves and others that they do not have celiac disease, they will intentionally eat gluten, and then usually suffer greatly for it. They may then suppress their discomfort, minimizing its severity, or they may attribute it to a different condition.

The cheater in denial who is testing herself with gluten is playing with fire, and will likely learn quickly that the one she's hurting the most is herself. With many kids, this "testing process" is just what the doctor ordered to *confirm* the diagnosis!

3. Just Doesn't Care

There are some people who just don't care. They don't care that they are doing significant damage to themselves internally. They don't care that they suffer gastrointestinal distress. It's more important to them that they be like everyone else, or that they not be inconvenienced with the dietary restrictions that go along with celiac disease.

These kids are going to cheat. The best you can do is continue to educate your child about the harm gluten is doing to her body, and hope that it's just a phase. Sometimes having a doctor discuss celiac disease with her is effective, since some kids are more likely to believe something if it doesn't come from their parents. Doctors hold a little more credibility than parents. (Sadly, with some kids at some ages, just about *anyone* is more credible than parents!) Even if your doctor can't convince your child of the importance of sticking to the diet, don't give up. Most kids do, eventually, learn to care.

4. Curious about Foods She's Never Tasted

It's very common for kids to be curious about what "the other kind" of food tastes like, especially if it has been a long time since they've had anything with gluten in it. These kids will sneak a little taste every now and then, but generally return to their strict adherence to a gluten-free diet, especially when they get that not-so-subtle reminder of how "the other kind" of food makes them feel.

5. Defeated

Kids and grown-ups alike fall into this category from time to time. These people feel that it's too hard to be 100 percent gluten-free. They figure if they're going to be getting a little gluten, they might as well be getting a lot, and they tend to be some of the worst cheaters of all.

5- to 12-Year-Olds: Armed and Dangerous

Kids this age tend to make a lot of mistakes in selecting "safe" foods. It's not that they're intentionally cheating. It's actually because they know too much. They know, for instance, that they can eat marshmallows. But what they don't always know, or conveniently choose to forget (in the case of the ten- to twelve-year-olds), is that they can't eat *all* marshmallows. The best you can do is talk to them when they make mistakes; explain how they can make a better decision in the future; and remind them that if they don't know for sure, they shouldn't eat it.

Dealing with Cheaters

Because they have minds, hands, and mouths of their own, you're not going to be able to stop a cheater who wants to cheat. But there are some things you can do that might help.

1. Make Sure Your Child Understands the Consequences

Don't preach, don't lecture, and whatever you do, don't nag. But make sure your child has a clear understanding that even the most minute traces of gluten can cause damage. Even if it's just licking a postage stamp or envelope—cheating can cause harm to her body.

2. Explain That 100 Percent Gluten-Free Is Unrealistic

If your child is feeling defeated by the diet, it may be that she's discouraged that every now and then she inadvertently gets some gluten, and can't seem to maintain 100 percent gluten-free status. She needs to know that's okay. No one can be 100 percent gluten-free all the time, because accidents do happen. Explain that all she can do is try her hardest to adhere to the diet, and that you're proud of her high expectations and discipline.

3. Encourage Her to Ask about "Normal" Foods

A lot of kids are curious about what "normal" food tastes like, especially when they have been on a gluten-free diet for a long time.

When your child asks, "What does your pizza taste like?" it might be tempting to say, "Oh, it's not as good as yours." Don't compare. First of all, your child won't believe you, and you'll lose all credibility. Secondly, most likely you'll be lying, and parents don't do that well. Rather than comparing, *tell* her what it tastes like! Try, though, to describe tastes that just happen to be in her pizza, too. Like the tomato sauce, the cheese, the pepperoni— she won't realize this at a conscious level, but subconsciously she'll be thinking, "Yeah, that's what I like about my pizza, too!"

Make sure your child feels comfortable asking about your food when she is curious. Some kids are so perceptive and sensitive to *your* feelings that they don't want to make you feel guilty, or feel sorry for them. So they just don't ask. But all kids on a restricted diet wonder about the foods they can't have, so make sure they feel as though you "can handle it."

Part of making sure your child feels that she can talk to you about her feelings requires that you be honest with her. Don't try to hide the big hot pretzel behind your back when she walks into the room. Unless your family is 100 percent gluten-free, she knows that other people eat gluten. If you hide it, and especially if you get caught hiding it, she'll feel that you're trying to spare her from feeling bad that she can't have something—and she'll draw the conclusion that she must be, in fact, missing out on something good.

4. Get Annual Blood Tests

Most doctors will tell you that your child should have the gluten antibody blood test annually, just to make sure she isn't inadvertently getting gluten in her diet. (See Chapter Twenty-Two.) In many cases, the annual testing is covered by standard indemnity, HMO, and PPO health plans. While annual testing is a good idea simply from a health maintenance standpoint, it has an additional benefit if you have a cheater on your hands. If you start the annual testing early, she will come to expect the test, and she'll know that she's going to get caught if she's cheating.

Don't use the blood test as a threat. If you suspect she's cheating, it might be tempting to threaten her with a blood test to see for sure. It's really better to let her know that the tests are part of an ongoing annual check-up, as recommended by your physician. Let the doctor be the fall guy!

It's Never Okay to Cheat

But it's her birthday! Isn't it okay for her to have just one teeny tiny bite of "regular" cake? Nope. For one thing, any parent who has made the mistake of saying, "Okay, just this once" knows that children have a special processor in their ears that translates that to, "Okay, any time you want." Rare is the child who thinks to herself, "Gee, I'd really like to have that, but Mommy said 'just this once,' so I'm not even going to ask again." Yeah, right. It might start as a little birthday treat, and next thing you know they'll be pointing out that Fridays are special days, too.

> "We're really good about sticking to the diet, and I know Derek never cheats. But he won first place in the science fair, and the judges gave out cupcakes to the top three winners to congratulate them. We thought maybe just this once it would be okay for him to have just a little. After all, we're so good most of the time."
> —Natalie G.

More importantly, from a health standpoint, that teeny tiny bite of cake is poison to your child's system. And psychologically, you're sending a hugely conflicting message to your child if you allow gluten "for special treats." You've told her how bad it is for her body; to allow an indulgence for a special occasion is like saying, "It's your birthday, so I'll let you harm your body and suffer the discomfort for several days in celebration. But just this once."

Do As I Say, Not As I Do

If you're on a special diet and you cheat, should you tell your child about how you cheated and suffered the consequences in order to illustrate why she shouldn't cheat? No! For one thing, you'll never possibly be able to articulate the consequences you suffered. Did you gain a few pounds when you cheated on a weight loss diet? Did you suffer a blood sugar imbalance on a diet to control diabetes? No matter what consequences you suffered, your child won't be able to empathize.

Again, kids have some special processor in their ears that translates our grown-up language into something they'd rather hear. If you say, "I cheated on my diet, and it took me months to heal" what they hear is, "I cheated on my diet, but it was no big deal." After all, what they see is the same old mom or dad. They can't tell if you gained a few pounds or felt a diabetic drop in blood sugar. In fact,

Are There Any Real "Antidotes" to Gluten?

There have been claims recently that various enzymes will assist in the "breakdown" of gluten, and may therefore be helpful to people with celiac disease who accidentally or even intentionally ingest gluten.

One such product is called SerenAid, which claims to contain enzymes that completely break down the proteins in grains (gluten) and dairy products (casein). The manufacturers claim that SerenAid results in a more complete breakdown of casein and gluten molecules, minimizing the absorption of peptides and protein fragments through the intestinal lining into the blood stream.

As tempting as it may be to use a product like this as an "antidote" to gluten, be extremely wary. Joseph A. Murray, M.D., of the Mayo Clinic says, "There is no evidence that it (SerenAid) will prevent the damaging effects of gluten in people with celiac disease. It is unlikely that it would be so efficient as to get rid of all of the gluten that has been swallowed. I would not recommend it as a treatment for celiac disease."

to them you seem perfectly fine, so the obvious conclusion now that you've admitted you cheated is that it must not have done any harm at all!

Tattling on the Cheater

No one likes a tattletale. But I think most parents agree that when it's a matter of safety, we need to hear about it. So what should you do if your child eats gluten and a sibling tells on her?

It depends on whether the act was intentional or an accident. If it was intentional, you should let the tattletale know that it was a good thing to tell you about it, and deal with your little cheater as you feel appropriate. But if it was an accident and little sister felt a need to tattle, it probably indicates that your child with celiac disease was not going to tell you on her own. That's a good chance for you to talk with her about how important it is for her to let you know when she's made a mistake, and that you aren't going to punish her. Unfortunately, she'll be dealing with punishment of her own.

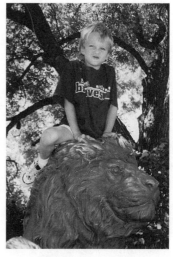

19

Gluten-Free or Not Gluten-Free
Why Is There A Question?

"I've been in contact with a few different support organizations, and they're not saying the same thing. One group says something is gluten-free, and the other says it isn't because there could be cross-contamination or trace amounts of gluten. How do I know which view is right?"
—Marti W.

If you're doing any networking or research on the Internet, you have likely heard varying opinions on the gluten-free status of many different foods. This is a hot potato issue in the celiac community.

It seems as though there should be a simple test for determining whether or not foods contain gluten. But there's not. In fact, different celiac organizations, medical professionals, and experts on celiac disease all seem to have differing opinions concerning several substances. Some of these include:

- Oats
- Canola oil
- Vinegar
- Vanilla
- Wheat starch
- Maltodextrin
- Monosodium glutamate (MSG)
- Caramel coloring

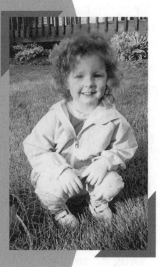

Although I have my own personal beliefs about whether or not these substances are gluten-free, at this time nobody can say with 100 percent assurance whether they are or not. (The

A Note on Oats

There is a raging controversy over whether or not oats truly contain gluten. Currently, evidence seems to indicate that the toxicity in pure oats is low, if it exists at all. The problem seems to be in finding uncontaminated oats. If it were *my* gut at risk, I might consider a "test" of oats, since there is, in fact, some strong evidence indicating it does not contain gluten. However, since it is my *child* involved, I have decided not to put him at risk.

exceptions are vinegar, vanilla, and canola, all of which have been determined to be safe for people with celiac disease after it is distilled—even if it is derived from a gluten-containing source.) The most prudent and practical thing for you to do is research the subjects yourself, and draw your own conclusions.

As you become more familiar with the diet, and which foods do or do not seem to bother your child, you will be able to make your own decisions on these controversial items. In the meantime, it's important to understand some of the reasons for the controversy on this subject.

Contamination

Most of the controversy revolves around the issue of contamination. Is the food product that appears to be gluten-free actually contaminated in some way with gluten?

Contamination can occur in otherwise gluten-free food items in a variety of ways:

- **Preparation:** Gluten-free foods are prepared with the same utensils, on the same cooking surfaces, or in the same "medium" (such as oil) as gluten-containing foods.
- **Processing:** When commercial products are processed, they are generally on what is referred to as a "line," which is usually a type of conveyor belt that physically moves the product through its production cycle. Sometimes a gluten-containing product is processed on the line right next to a gluten-free product. Other times, the same line is used for both types of products. While this may seem at first as though it would "obviously" turn a gluten-free product into a celiac response waiting to happen, it's important to note that the Food and Drug Administration requires all food manu-

"My brother did some research on celiac disease and said that we shouldn't let our son eat the fries at McDonald's because they might be fried in the same oil as something with gluten in it. Do I really need to be concerned about how the food is cooked?"
—Leanna W.

facturers and ingredient suppliers to follow careful guidelines called Good Manufacturing Practices (GMP) when cleaning equipment.

- **Bulk Bins:** The bulk bins at grocery stores can be contaminated because they sit close to one another, and people may dig into several different bins with the same scoop.
- **Growing Grains:** Sometimes gluten-free grains will be grown in fields close to gluten-containing grains. Some people believe that cross-contamination can occur while the plants are still growing.

So, how seriously do you take the issue of contamination? I'm not touching that one with a ten-foot pole. It's a personal decision that boils down to: How crazy do you want to make yourself?

Of course, you need to be aware of the possibility of contamination, and make wise food choices. If you're at a fast-food restaurant and they have the fries cooking in the same oil as the onion rings, you might want to think twice about those fries. Not that the oil itself would *necessarily* cause a problem, but surely there are pieces of the onion-ring breading floating around, and it's pretty likely that they could make their way into your fry basket.

How Perfect Do We Have to Be?

Just how stringent you need to be in making decisions about what is gluten-free and what isn't is another controversial subject, with vocal and knowledge-able advocates at both ends of the spectrum. Of course, without a doubt, you should be as diligent about keeping your child as gluten-free as possible.

Having said that, no one is perfect. Don't expect yourself to be, and certainly don't expect your child to be. Don't beat yourself or your child up over the mistakes that will be made.

One of the most positive, constructive approaches I've heard comes from Ann Whelan, editor and publisher of the *Gluten-Free Living* newsletter and a person with celiac disease herself. The following is an excerpt from an editorial she published in the March/April 1999 edition.

"Let's stop worrying that the next potential trace of possible gluten that might find its way into our bodies is going to kill us. Unscientific exaggerations like this scare and mislead people, make them depressed and even cause many to cheat on the grounds that it makes no difference since we all live in a gluten-filled world and are likely doomed anyway.

"By the time we've considered the possibility of cross-contamination, whether or not distillation actually eliminates any trace of gluten, and how foods are processed, it seems like there's nothing left that we can feed our daughter. How perfect do we have to be?"
—Ted D.

"Yes, we all need to stay as gluten-free as possible, but responsibly gluten-free. Fearing a scientifically unmeasurable, theoretically impossible but not proven-beyond-a-skeptical-celiac-doubt molecule of gliadin has an unhealthful paranoid tone to it. It's a bit like deciding to stay indoors in the dark when the sun is up once the words basal cell cancer enter your life."

20

Celiac Teens
Not Just Gluten Intolerant, But Parent Intolerant, Too

"Kary was diagnosed at age three, and did fine with the diet—until she turned thirteen. Now it seems she's always threatening to go off the diet, using it almost as a weapon against me. It used to be so much easier. I wonder what happened."
—Larry M.

If your child was diagnosed well before adolescence, you may have just been sailing along with a child who took full control of her diet and never had the desire to cheat or tempt gluten-laden fate. Then adolescence hits, and suddenly she's heading for the pizza parlor for "the real thing" and telling you there's nothing you can do about it.

As though the challenges of dealing with teenagers weren't enough, dealing with teenagers who have the dietary restrictions that go along with celiac disease can be—well, let's just say "difficult" and leave it at that.

Perhaps some of you are thinking, *"My teenager is a dream and isn't going through* 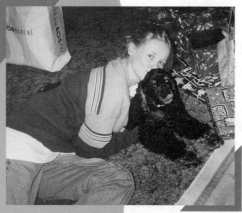 that typical teen rebellion that my friends talk about." Well, then you can skip this chapter—or maybe you'll want to read it for your "friends" who have typical teens. And then again, you could wait five minutes for your teen's next mood to hit.

The bottom line is that teens act differently because they *are* different. They experience immense physi-

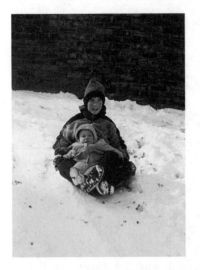

cal, intellectual, and emotional changes, all in a very short period of time. During this time they have amazing powers. They can transform themselves from Beaver Cleaver into Freddy Krueger in a matter of five minutes or less. They can turn a glorious family reunion into a scene from *The Exorcist* with one wrong word. They can interpret "Please clean up your room" as "I hate you, love your brother more, and wish you had never been born." Their emotional roller coasters would be the envy of any amusement park designer.

One of the most significant of all emotional changes is that they feel a sense of independence, power, and control over their bodies and their lives that they cannot ignore. Their lives transform from being dominated by their parents to being dominated by themselves. They forcefully and purposefully *push* their childhood behind—and pull away from their parents' grasp.

Letting G-g-g-g-go

Just as it's their job to grow up, it's *your* job to let go. I'm not sure if it's more difficult to let go because you're afraid they still need you, or because you're afraid they won't.

The hardest part of letting go at this point is that you can't let go completely. You have to find and then walk that fine line of letting go enough that they learn to conquer the world on their own, yet still maintain enough control that you are setting limits and confronting them with their undesirable behavior.

What this means to the parents of teens with celiac disease is that there *will* be times when they make "mistakes." And many times they *will* be intentional.

So, how do you respond to your child's blatant disregard for her body? You express your concern, and then you bite your tongue. She'll be expecting a lecture, so whatever you do, don't give her one. The beauty of this particular condition is that *she's* the one who will suffer most. And for a teenager, I can't think of a worse punishment than to be slammed with a bad case of odiferous flatulence accompanied by a good old dose of diarrhea.

Acceptance = Happiness

To a teen, happiness comes from being accepted by your friends. So it is no wonder that celiac teens have a difficult time dealing with their very special diet. After all, at a point in their lives when they judge one another on the most trivial discrepancies from "the norm," it's just not cool to be eating pizza made on a corn tortilla.

How their friends respond to their diet can either make it incredibly easy for them to deal with, or incredibly difficult. While most of us assume that peers would make this period difficult on a child with celiac disease, Joan Wade of Sylvan Borders Farm Gluten-Free Products has a refreshingly positive perspective.

"I spent twenty-five years as a teacher before I changed careers. I have always felt that the easiest age group to help with an adjustment to a gluten-free diet would be the middle school students. They are so bonded as an age group. They share clothes, hairbrushes, tapes, CD's, etc. I am sure if a child had to be on a gluten-free diet, a gang of friends would go grocery shopping with her and read every label in the store. The press and the community as a whole don't see the caring that exists between students. I just thought I would share this perspective with you as a person reaching out to children who previously spent so many years in a classroom with them."

The Teen Who Is Newly Diagnosed

Imagine—your teen's body has changed to the point that she truly does not recognize herself anymore. She wants to be grown up, but she wants to be taken care of. She has school, friends, and responsibilities to juggle, and parents who won't get off her back. The one thing she has full control over is her body. And then that's taken away, because she's being told she can't eat *anything* she and her friends used to eat.

Because of all the inherent stress factors in being a teenager, diagnosis at this point could just be too much for her to handle on her own. If your teen seems to be having a difficult time accepting the condition, seek counseling immediately, preferably from a professional who understands both teens and dietary restrictions (e.g., diabetes). Most pediatricians will be able to refer you to a knowledgeable mental health professional.

Sometimes it helps for teens to talk to teens. The celiac community is very supportive, and if you ask, there will be teens who will contact yours and let her know she's not alone. Contact your local chapter of a national celiac support organization. If you don't have the number of a local chapter, call the national organization and see what they can do to help. It might also be helpful for your teen to subscribe to the celiac LISTSERV, or for someone to submit a query to the LISTSERV to see if any parents would ask their teen to contact yours. (See the Resource Guide for information on the celiac LISTSERV as well as celiac support organizations.)

Using Celiac Disease to Get What She Wants (AKA Manipulation)

Picture yourself in the following situation: Missy (oops, it's Melissa now) wants to go to Tara's house on a weeknight.

"Mom, can I go to Tara's house to listen to CDs tonight?"

"No, Missy, uh, Melissa. It's a Tuesday night, and you know we don't allow you to go out on a school night."

"But Mom, *everyone else* gets to go out on a school night!"

"I said no. We have rules in this house, and that's one of them."

"But (tears beginning to flow on command) Tara is the only one who understands about me having celiac disease. She's the only one who doesn't make fun of me. Just today, Karen and Joanne were calling me a freak because I eat such stupid stuff. They said my muffin looked like a pile of sawdust glued together. No one else understands! *You* don't understand! Tara is the only one who understands. *She* makes me feel okay about it, and I could sure use *her* support right now. . . ."

Bullseye. Right smack dab in the middle of your heart. Button numero-uno, she pulls the sympathy card.

The best way to avoid being vulnerable to the manipulation game is to be prepared for the attack. Remember the *real* point of the conversation, and stick to your rules. Obviously, her condition and Tara's sympathetic nature have nothing to do with whether or not you allow your kids to go out on a school night. So, as much as they try to derail you by honing in on your own feelings of guilt or sympathy, be resolute in your stand, and put the discussion back on track.

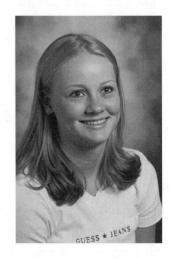

Dating and Parties

As though a first date isn't stressful enough, teens with celiac disease may think they have reason to be especially nervous. If the date will be at a restaurant, should they mention their condition to their date? What about when it comes time to have dinner with her boyfriend's parents?

There are no right and wrong ways for parents to help their teens with these kinds of feelings. As a parent, however, you should be aware that dating may be more anxiety-provoking for your child, and you should make it clear that you are always available to discuss these things with her. Hopefully, you've been talking with your child all along about how real friends treat their friends (see Chapter

Fourteen). This may be a good time to remind her that someone who is worth knowing will not judge her by her diet.

While you're having "the talk," don't forget to talk to your teen about drinking alcohol. Regardless of your personal views on underage drinking, you and your child should both know and discuss the fact that beer and many other alcoholic beverages are loaded with gluten.

Hormones and the "Honeymoon Period"

Celiac disease does a strange thing during adolescence. It actually appears to "go away." In fact, celiac disease never "goes away," and children do not outgrow it. But usually around the onset of puberty, most likely due to the many hormonal changes, celiacs who eat gluten no longer feel the effects—at least not as much as they once did. Specialists refer to this as the "honeymoon phase."

> "Sophie was showing signs of celiac disease for a few years, but when she turned twelve, they seemed to go away. We just figured she outgrew it."
> —Sheldon T.

This is a very dangerous phase. Without the diarrhea and cramping, teens figure it must be okay to eat gluten, and they go crazy making up for lost gluten-eating time! But the gluten molecules are still doing harm to the small intestine, laying the groundwork for severe consequences down the road.

Denial—among kids, of course, but also among parents—is very common during the honeymoon phase. Eager to believe that their kids don't have celiac disease, parents begin to suspect a misdiagnosis. After all, look at them now! They can eat *anything*, and they feel just fine! It's a false and dangerous sense of security. If you truly suspect a misdiagnosis, you may want to have the antibody screening (blood test) done. But remember, to obtain accurate antibody results, your child must be eating a gluten-containing diet for at least a few weeks. (See Chapter Twenty-Two for more information on testing.)

The honeymoon period generally ends in the late teenage years or early twenties. At that point, if the child has been gluten-free, there will be little or no change in her condition. She's gluten-free, and except for the difficulties experienced as a result of raging hormones, she should be a healthy, normal teen (is that an oxymoron?).

But if she has been eating gluten with no apparent symptoms, thanks to the honeymoon period, she may begin to experience the discomfort that most people with celiac disease feel when they eat gluten.

You might think that many diagnoses are made during young adulthood as teens are coming off their honeymoon period. Surprisingly, while there are more diagnoses made in the early twenties than, say, the mid-teens, it is not as commonly diagnosed at this time as one might think.

There are a few reasons for this paradox. One is that at this age, young adults are beginning to leave home to venture out on their own. They may be distracted by the many other exciting things going on in their lives, such as finding an apartment, beginning a career, and becoming involved in serious relationships. They may not even notice their discomfort.

Or, they may feel the symptoms of celiac disease, but chalk them up to the new stresses they are facing. Beginning a life on their own, they may also be hesitant to seek medical help because of the costs involved.

For whatever reason, many people who begin to feel symptoms after breaking out of the honeymoon phase ignore them, and even become used to them. These people often blame their discomfort on a presumed lactose intolerance, stress, irritable bowel syndrome, or some other ambiguous condition. They will usually suffer for years before seeking medical advice, and will be diagnosed later in life—if at all.

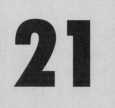

What Causes Celiac Disease?

People often ask what "causes" celiac disease. Nothing "causes" it, although something *may* trigger it. People with celiac disease have a "genetic predisposition" for developing celiac disease. That is, they carry a gene or genes that *may* result in celiac disease under some circumstances, but not others.

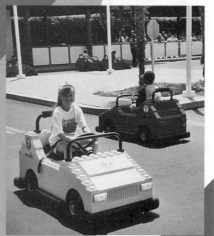

Recent research has indicated that celiac disease is *multigenetic*. This means that it's more complex than being simply a "dominant" trait, passed on by one parent or a "recessive" trait, passed on by both parents. There are several genes involved, each of which may have different strengths of expression.

The important thing to note is that if your child has celiac disease, it's because the disorder "runs" in one or both sides of the family. Often after a child is diagnosed, parents will realize that, interestingly, Grandma had lymphoma (cancer), or Grandpa never did eat bread because he said it made him feel bad, Dad feels lousy after drinking a beer, or someone in the family was told at some point that he had a wheat "allergy." It is likely that many of the family members have had celiac disease, but were never diagnosed.

Genetics don't tell the whole story, though. We know this because identical twins, genetically the same in every way, do not always both get celiac disease. In fact, in "only" 70-75 percent of identical twin sets do both twins have celiac disease; in the other 25-30 percent, only one of the twins has it. The non-genetic factors are not yet known, but certain viruses or stress triggers are suspected.*

What Triggers Celiac Disease?

Since celiac disease is a genetic disorder, the tendency to acquire celiac disease is present at birth. It is not yet understood why people get the damage (disease) at any particular age. Perhaps an infection causes initial damage to the intestine, allowing the immune system to recognize gliadin as "foreign." This may set the disease process going.

Some children exhibit severe symptoms soon after gluten is introduced into their diet. Others show mild symptoms in early childhood, but the symptoms seem to mysteriously "disappear" between the ages of six (or so) until after puberty. This is referred to as a "honeymoon period," and no one is quite sure why this occurs. Tolerance to gluten, or lack of symptoms in adolescence, is very common.

Yet others show absolutely no symptoms until their twenties, thirties, forties, or later. It is thought that a "trigger" of some sort eventually prompts an individual to get the disease. Then there may be another trigger that results in the actual symptoms of the disease. Triggers can include a virus, pregnancy, surgery or other physical trauma to the body, or stress. Sometimes there just isn't an explanation for what triggered the symptoms to appear—they're just there. And, probably most commonly, the symptoms were there all along, but they were ignored, masked, or misdiagnosed as irritable bowel syndrome, lactose intolerance, gas, or other benign and common conditions. Often people get used to "feeling lousy," chronic fatigue, or a variety of gastrointestinal discomforts.

What Happens Once Celiac Disease is Triggered?

Celiac disease is an *autoimmune disorder.* An autoimmune disorder is a general term for disorders in which the body produces immune reactions against itself,

---

* *Questions and Answers on HLA Typing and Celiac Disease,* Version 1.3. Copyright Michael Jones, Bill Elkus, Jim Lyles, and Lisa Lewis, 1995, 1996, 1997—All rights reserved worldwide.

resulting in tissue injury. The immune system is a complicated network of cells and cell components (called *molecules*) that normally work to defend the body and eliminate infections caused by bacteria, viruses, and other invading microbes. When someone has an autoimmune disease, the immune system mistakenly attacks itself, targeting the cells, tissues, and organs of that person's own body.

Most immune system cells are white blood cells, of which there are many types. Lymphocytes are one type of white blood cell, and two major classes of lymphocytes are *T-cells* and *B-cells*. T-cells are critical immune system cells that help to destroy infected cells and coordinate the overall immune response, fighting cold viruses and other external threats to the body. B-cells are best known for making antibodies.

In people with celiac disease, T-cells in the intestines respond specifically to something in gluten, mistaking gluten for a substance that needs to be eliminated from the body. To be precise, the T-cells react against the portion of gluten that is linked to a protein in the human body called tissue transglutaminase. This results in the T-cells— which usually *fight off* damage to the body—causing damage to the villi.

Because celiac disease is an autoimmune disorder, you may be concerned that your child's immune system is compromised. In fact, your child's immune system is *over*active, not underactive. But while your child is chronically ill from celiac disease, he will have more trouble fighting infections. This may be due to poor nutrition. In addition, early in the disease the spleen does not function well. This makes people more susceptible to certain bacterial infections.

Is Celiac Disease an Allergy? NO!

Many people refer to celiac disease as an allergy. It's *not* an allergy, but an autoimmune disorder, as explained above.

I believe it's dangerous for people to think that celiac disease is an allergy. Some parents, believing it is an allergy, will feed their children gluten, followed by an antihistamine to "counteract the allergic reaction." Others believe that allergies can be "overcome" through a desensitization process of gradually introducing the allergen back into the diet. (There is controversy over whether this is, in fact, true.) If, however, someone slowly introduces gluten into the diet of child with celiac disease, it is like feeding him poison. Slowly. And finally, people *can* outgrow an allergy. But no matter how hard you wish, your child will not outgrow celiac disease.

If you are interested in the physiological difference between an allergy and an autoimmune disorder, read on. The rest of you can skip ahead! Technically, the difference is this: with an allergy, an allergen (the substance you're allergic to) is detected by the B-cells in your blood. The B-cells see that allergen as an enemy, and produce an antibody that is very specifically designed to fight that allergen.

In the case of allergies, the antibody produced is called IgE (immunoglobulin E). Histamine is then released. Histamine is the chemical that causes us to feel so bad when we have an allergic reaction. The reaction generally occurs quite quickly.

In celiac disease, on the other hand, there is no release of IgE when the body detects gluten. The reaction occurs much more slowly, so symptoms can be delayed by as much as a day or two (which is why it can be difficult to pinpoint the food someone can't tolerate). And, as explained above, the reaction is really against a part of the body itself, and gluten is just the trigger to that reaction. Another difference is that the effects of gluten on someone with celiac disease are cumulative, causing more and more damage to the villi every time it is ingested.

Could Other Family Members Have It?

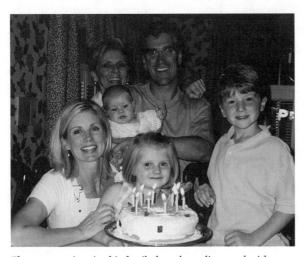

Three generations in this family have been diagnosed with celiac disease.

Absolutely. Celiac disease is a genetic condition, which means someone in your child's biological ancestry passed it down. It also means that relatives may have it—and they may not even know it. The more closely related someone is to your child with celiac disease, the more likely it is that they have it or will develop symptoms. There is an estimated 10-30 percent incidence in first-degree (direct) relatives (meaning parents, children, and siblings).* Many (estimates range from 10 to 50 percent) first-degree relatives have asymptomatic celiac disease, which means they show no symptoms.** It is important to remember, however, that while people have varying degrees of *symptoms*, there is no such thing as having a "milder" case of celiac disease. Either you have it or you don't.

The next chapter explains the diagnostic process for anyone who is suspected of having celiac disease.

---

* "Familial Incidence of Celiac Disease," presented aboard Celiac Experience III, January 1994 by Joseph A. Murray, M.D.

** Karoly Horvath, M.D., as written in *Gluten-Free Living Magazine,* January/February 1999.

22 The Diagnosis
Tests, Tests, and More Tests

Celiac disease is grossly underdiagnosed, especially in the United States. Recent figures indicate that as many as 1 in 150 Americans has celiac disease, whereas only about 1 in 2000 is diagnosed. That means that hundreds of thousands of people are undiagnosed, feeling lousy, sometimes even suffering grave health consequences, and not knowing why.

Often physicians misdiagnose people with celiac disease as having a variety of other disorders such as a reaction to antibiotics, the flu, and even chronic disorders such as irritable bowel syndrome, Crohn's disease, allergies, unexplained failure to thrive, or chronic fatigue syndrome.

Misdiagnosis can be dangerous and even life-threatening. People with celiac disease who continue to eat gluten become malnourished, deficient in important nutrients, anemic, lethargic, and most definitely uncomfortable if gastrointestinal distress is one of their symptoms. They are 40 to 100 times more likely to develop intestinal lymphoma, a type of cancer. Even infertility problems have been attributed to undiagnosed celiac disease.

Diagnosing Celiac Disease

The procedures involved in diagnosing celiac disease are relatively straight-forward and simple. Getting your doctor to perform those procedures and arrive at a diagnosis can be the tough part. Most of us parents have consulted at *least* one pediatrician who brushed off our child's symptoms with a myriad of possible explanations: it's the antibiotics you're giving her for her ear infection; it's the flu; it's a reaction to something she ate. Whatever the excuse, they hand you a sheet of paper with the B.R.A.T. diet, and tell you to go home and wait it out. Diarrhea tends to be difficult to get rid of, they tell you. Many doctors even joke about how cute toddlers look with a big, round belly.

One problem is that many primary care pediatricians are not aware of celiac disease. Often they'll tell you that what you *perceive* to be problems—irritability, a distended belly, diarrhea—are "normal" for children. They may dismiss you with the patronizing advice that you should relax; nothing is wrong with your child. Even when asked directly about celiac disease, or told that celiac disease runs in the family, many pediatricians refuse to test for it. They may tell you that because your child is growing at a "normal" pace, is normal height and weight, she couldn't have celiac disease. This is *not* true!

If you reach an impasse with your pediatrician, you have four options: 1) find a new doctor (we went through *four*, because our instincts told us that something was definitely wrong with our child, even though three doctors in-sisted that the symptoms should be ignored); 2) educate your doctor (not all physicians are amenable to this, but if you have one who is, you're in good hands); 3) ask to be referred to a specialist; or 4) and this is not truly an accept-able option—trust that the doctor is right, and hope that your child is not get-ting worse with every bite of cracker.

If your child has symptoms, or even if there are no symptoms but celiac disease runs in your family, it is absolutely imperative that you insist on having your child tested. Change doctors if yours refuses, but don't stop until you suc-ceed in finding someone who will test your child.

Finding a Competent Specialist

A gastroenterologist is the specialist who is qualified to diagnose and super-vise treatment of celiac disease. Gastroenterologists are medical doctors with training and expertise in disorders of the digestive tract. In the case of celiac disease in children, the specialist is a *pediatric* gastroenterologist, sometimes re-ferred to as a pediatric "G.I."

Don't let the specialist intimidate you. It's important for you to ask a lot of questions to make sure your child's health is truly in the hands of someone who understands celiac disease. Just because the doctor is a gastroenterologist does *not* mean he knows about celiac disease.

If you feel your gastroenterologist is not truly knowledgeable, request a new one immediately. Proper diagnosis and ongoing monitoring must be done by a competent specialist, and you have the right to ask as many questions as it takes for you to feel comfortable with your doctor's knowledge on the subject.

Some questions to ask your doctor:

- How many patients with celiac disease have you seen? (It's okay if he hasn't seen many, or even *any*, as long as you feel he truly understands the disease, and has kept up with recent research.)
- How many do you currently see? (Again, it's okay if the answer is "none." He can be perfectly competent without having seen any.)
- What is your knowledge of celiac disease? (This is an intentionally open-ended question.)
- What sub-specialties do you have? (Many gastroenterologists sub-specialize in malabsorption—this is a good indication that your doctor is knowledgeable about celiac disease.)
- What form of diagnosis do you use?
- Don't be smug, but tactfully ask questions that you know the answer to (don't let him know you already know the answer). Unfortunately, not all doctors keep up with the latest research. The last few years have been revolutionary in the study of celiac disease, and you want to make sure your doctor is keeping up with the literature. Some questions you might want to ask are:
  - Do people outgrow celiac disease? (The answer should be no.)
  - How rare is it? (If he indicates that it's *very* rare, or even somewhat rare, you'll know he's not up to date. It's okay to ask him statistics. Remember, the right answer is approximately as many as 1 in 150 to 250 people.)
  - What causes celiac disease?
  - If one of my children has it, how likely is it that my other child will have it? (The answer is that there is about a 30 percent chance.)
  - Is it okay to have just a little gluten every once in awhile?

Testing Procedures

There are three accepted methods for diagnosing celiac disease, although some are considered to substantiate a positive diagnosis more than others. The simplest, least expensive, and least invasive diagnostic tool is the serum (blood) antibody test. The "gold standard" for confirming a diagnosis of celiac disease is a small bowel biopsy (sometimes a series of biopsies). The following sections detail these testing procedures.

Serological (Blood) Testing

Looking for specific antibodies in the blood (serum) is a very helpful way to screen people for celiac disease because the test is so easy. The results indicate whether someone is likely (or not likely) to have the disease, but cannot confirm the diagnosis. They are a good first step to determining who should undergo further, more invasive testing.

Sometimes doctors don't mention an important detail: it is essential that your child be on a gluten-*containing* diet for at least six months prior to testing. Without gluten in the diet, there will not be an antibody response, and the test will be inconclusive.

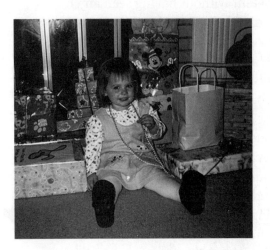

It is also important to note that a negative screening does not mean your child doesn't have celiac disease. Several factors can affect the results of the screening, and because some of the readings can be subjective, further testing may be required.

Serological testing is also a good tool *after* a positive diagnosis of celiac disease is made through endoscopic testing (see below). In fact, your child should be tested annually to make sure her diet is, in fact, 100 percent gluten-free. Sometimes the blood screening will reveal elevated antibody levels, and you will discover that something in your child's diet that you *thought* was gluten-free, in fact does contain gluten.

The purpose of doing the blood test for celiac disease is to check for the presence of antibodies in the bloodstream. Specifically, your child's doctor will be looking for the following antibodies: anti-gliadin, anti-endomysium, anti-reticulin, and anti-transglutaminase. Two of the antibodies that the doctor is looking for respond to gliadin; they fight it as though it were an enemy of the body. These antibodies are called antigliadin (AGA) IgA and IgG.

Sometimes antireticulin (ARA) antibodies are evaluated. The amount of ARA in the blood correlates to the degree of intestinal damage. The tests for ARA are less sensitive than other blood tests, however, so they are considered less valuable than other serological tests. The tests for anti-transglutaminase IgA and IgG are also done less frequently, as they are relatively new and are just available in a few labs.

Another antibody that doctors look for in diagnosing celiac disease is called antiendomysial (EmA). The immune system of people with celiac disease makes these antibodies in reaction to the ingestion of gluten, and they "attack" the endomysium, which is connective tissue found around the smooth muscle cells of the intestine. EmA is very specific for celiac disease. That means that if someone does *not* have celiac disease, she will likely have a negative test result. It also has an extremely high "positive predictive

Tissue Transglutaminase (tTG)

Tissue Transglutaminase IgA and IgG is a relatively new blood test that has recently been introduced to detect celiac disease. The testing procedure itself is much more objective than other serological tests for celiac disease, so the results are considered to be more certain. Most of the labs listed in the Resource Guide are now doing tTG testing. According to Joseph Murray, M.D., of the Mayo Clinic, the tTG may replace the gliadin and endomysial testing in many circumstances.

value." This means that patients with a positive test for EmA likely have celiac disease. ***The EmA antibodies are the most important in diagnosing celiac disease.***

Antireticulin (ARA) antibodies correlate to the degree of intestinal damage, and may also be evaluated in the serological exams for celiac disease.

Get all of the tests. While blood tests cannot be used to make a definitive diagnosis, they can be very useful in making a probable diagnosis. But serological testing is only useful if all of the tests are done (sometimes doctors will order only one of the antibodies to be tested).

Choosing a Competent Lab to Do the Tests

Your child's blood can be drawn in the pediatrician's office, or at a lab associated with the office. But where the *testing* is done is extremely important. Very often, these tests are done improperly, even by reputable labs.

There are two reasons it is so important to have tests done at a competent lab. First, for the test to provide meaningful results, it must be validated using a large number of clinical documented subjects. (That is, the lab needs to have done many of these blood tests so they know how to interpret test results.) In addition, two of the tests, endomysial and reticulin, are complicated tests where the readings are subjective. One competent technician may read it differently than another one does. But lab personnel experienced with reading these particular tests will have done so in the past, and will be more likely to provide an accurate assessment.

The tests can be expensive ($250 - $350), and some insurance companies will not cover testing if you request a particular lab. Check with one of the national celiac organizations listed in the Resource Guide. Sometimes they know of university studies being done, where you can have the tests done for free.

There are several labs that have excellent reputations for celiac testing. They are listed in the Resource Guide at the back of this book.

Celiac Antibodies

Antigliadin antibody (AGA)
  IgG
  IgA
Antiendomysial antibody (EMA)
Antireticulin antibody (ARA)
Antitransglutaminase antibody (tTG)
  IgA
  IgG

	% of Sensitivity	% Specificity	Predictive Value (Pos) %	Predictive Value (Neg) %
tTG (human) IgA	98%	99%		
tTG (human) IgG	99%	92%		
EmA	97%	98%	97%	98%
ARA	65%	100%	100%	72%
AGA IgG	88%	92%	88%	92%
AGA IgA	52%	94%	87%	74%

Definitions:

Sensitivity: The probability of a positive test result in a patient with disease.

Specificity: The probability of negative test result in a patient without disease.

Positive predictive value: The probability of disease in a patient with positive test result.

Negative predictive value: The probability of no disease in a patient with negative test result.

EMA-IgA/tTG	AGA-Ig	AGA-IgG	Interpretation
+	+	+	CD almost certain
+	+	-	CD almost certain
+	-	+	CD almost certain
+	-	-	CD almost certain
-	+	+	CD probable
-	+	-	CD less likely
-	-	+	CD unlikely*
-	-	-	CD very unlikely

*These results need to be interpreted with care, as some patients with these results may actually have celiac disease.

The "Gold Standard" for Diagnosing Celiac Disease: Endoscopy/Biopsy

Most physicians agree that the most accurate form of diagnosis is a series of intestinal endoscopies to biopsy the small intestine. Your child will be sedated, either with "conscious sedation" or, more likely, "unconscious sedation" (general anesthesia). While there are some risks inherent in anesthesia itself, general anesthesia is a safer way to perform an endoscopy because your child is completely relaxed.

The pediatric gastroenterologist usually does the actual procedure. An anesthesiologist is also present. A tube (endoscope) is inserted through the mouth, and threaded to the small intestine. There, the doctor takes several tissue samples, and sends them to a lab for a biopsy. The lab inspects the villi to see if they have flattened out (mucosal atrophy), or are blunted. The biopsy itself is not painful, because there are no pain-sensitive nerves inside the small intestine.

Generally, the test is done first while your child is still very sick with symptoms or positive to the blood tests. It is important that your child is still on a gluten-containing diet at the time of the endoscopy. The expectation at that time is to see blunted, atrophied villi.

If the villi are, in fact, damaged, then it is presumed that there is a strong possibility of celiac disease. Your child is put on a gluten-free diet for several (usually three to six) months. In some cases, a second biopsy is then performed (expecting, of course, to see an improvement in the villi). In the past, this second biopsy was considered crucial. However, the recent international consensus is that one biopsy should be sufficient. If the child's symptoms then improve on a gluten-free diet and/or she tests negative to the blood tests after several months on the diet, most doctors would consider that proof enough that she has celiac disease.

Years ago, physicians generally recommended a third biopsy, for final confirmation. This was often referred to as the "challenge." The challenge involved putting the child back on gluten for a period of time (generally a month or two), and doing a third biopsy (expecting to see damaged villi again). Challenges are not performed very often anymore. If your doctor recommends one, be sure to ask him why. If he is questioning the diagnosis, ask him whether he reviewed the original biopsy. There is some evidence that challenges may actually be harmful to children.

While it *is* still considered the "gold standard" in diagnosing celiac disease, the biopsy does involve risks. There is a slight chance of internal injury, such as perforation of the bowel or excessive bleeding. Also, the sample of villi is small, and may not be representative of the entire small intestine. (This is why the doctor should take more than one piece from different areas of the duodenum.) Furthermore, it can be difficult to obtain a good sample and some physicians may not be as "good" as others. Interpretation of the results can be subjective, as well.

And finally, a "false negative" result can occur. In other words, a biopsy that comes back negative for celiac disease does not necessarily mean the patient doesn't have celiac disease.

Since the proper interpretation of the biopsy is necessary for diagnosis, it is crucial that the person interpreting it be very experienced in celiac disease. Sometimes the intestinal damage is so slight that only experienced eyes can recognize it. It's important to follow your instinct, and to press further with your doctor when you feel further testing or another opinion is warranted. And remember not to put your child on a gluten-free diet before having the biopsy done. If need be, you can try the diet *after* the biopsy if the results are not conclusive.

Genetic Testing: The HLA "Fingerprint"

We all have a "genetic fingerprint" called HLA (Human Leukocyte Antigens). Scott Yoder, M.D., explains that HLAs are proteins that protrude from the surface of cells, and are specific to each person. They allow the immune cells in the body to recognize things that belong to that person (and only that person). Immune cells bind (stick) to the HLA. If it's the "right" (i.e. "host") HLA, then the immune cells leave it alone. If it's "wrong" (i.e., transplanted from another person), then the immune cells initiate a response to the tissue and try to kill it. Because every person has a unique set of HLAs, they can be used in genetic testing to evaluate many different conditions.

Researchers are finding that certain types of HLA are especially prevalent in people with celiac disease. Certain genes within the HLA region of chromosome six are highly associated with the susceptibility to celiac disease, and appear to be necessary, but not sufficient, for the development of this condition. In other words, there is a strong genetic predisposition to develop celiac disease, but this predisposition alone is not enough for someone to develop celiac disease. To date, researchers have not been able to pinpoint the specific abnormal or mutated genes involved, although they are believed to lie in region "D" of MHC (Major Histocompatibility Complex) on the sixth chromosome.

You cannot have celiac disease if you do not have these genes. However, about 25 to 30 percent of people who do have the genes do not have celiac disease.

Genetic testing of the DNA extracted from your child's blood can determine the presence or absence of these HLA types. When some of these HLA types are found to be present, it can be an excellent way to confirm a diagnosis. It does not provide a diagnosis in and of itself, but it can be useful for people whose blood tests have come back ambiguous (high in some areas, low in others).

Remember, if your child turns out not to have genes compatible with having celiac disease, she cannot have the disorder. If she does have those genes, you cannot be positive that she has celiac disease, but further testing is definitely warranted because she is at risk. Genetic testing is expensive compared to the other blood tests and is not done in many labs, so you may have trouble getting your HMO or health insurance to agree to pay for it.

Other Tests That May Indicate Celiac Disease

There are other tests that can contribute to a confirmation of celiac disease.

Fatty Stool Test: Your doctor may ask you to closely examine your child's stool to see if it floats. What they're really looking for is the fat content. A high fat content, or positive fatty stool test, can occur in people with celiac disease, but may also occur in people with cystic fibrosis or pancreatic insufficiency.

Stools float for one of two reasons. *Steatorrhea* is a condition in which fat is not absorbed by the small intestine, so it is passed on in the stool. (In people with celiac disease, this is because the villi are blunted, therefore absorbing little or nothing.) A child with steatorrhea produces stool that is pale in color, floats, and leaves an oily film on the water surface. The second cause for stools floating is excessive gas. When a lot of gas is absorbed into the stool, it will float because of the air in it. This type of floating stool, however, is usually dark in color and does not leave an oily film on the surface of the water, so it is not quite the same as fatty stools seen in celiac disease.

Tests for Malabsorption: Your doctor may ask for other tests that can tell him whether your child has difficulties with malabsorption (due to celiac disease or another intestinal disorder) and how serious it is. He may order blood tests to measure the levels of: blood cells, albumin, cholesterol, glucose, calcium, phosphate, sodium, potassium, magnesium, zinc, and/or iron. These tests can provide an indirect proof that something is going on in your child's intestine.

Preparing Your Child for Testing: Honesty Is the Best Policy

It is important to talk honestly with your child about what to expect. Even the blood tests, which are really rather non-invasive and anti-climatic, are terrifying for most children (and parents!). The anticipation can put everyone on edge, and the labs are usually cold, sterile, impersonal, and less-than-inviting.

Blood Tests

If your child is having a blood test done, you may want to ask your doctor for a prescription for a topical anesthetic so your child won't feel the needle stick. About twenty minutes before the procedure, put some on both arms (sometimes they miss a vein in one arm and have to switch to the other one), and wrap plastic wrap over it to make sure it doesn't rub off.

Remember to think like kids do. After our son had blood drawn when he was four, we found out that he was mortified that they had taken so much. With a quivering lip and all the bravado he could muster, but with genuine fear for his life, he asked where we were going to find more blood to put back in. He was pretty sure they had drained him close to empty. It never occurred to us to explain beforehand that our bodies make blood to replace the stuff they take out, and that our bodies have *lots* more blood left anyway.

If your child is still young enough that she'll let you hold her, have her sit on your lap while the blood is being drawn. The phlebotomist (blood-draw-er) will put a tourniquet ("rubber band") on your child's arm. That's your cue to start distracting her with conversation, finger games with her other hand, or even a hand-held video game. Or, you may want to have her put the tourniquet on you first. This seems to be the scariest part of the procedure. If the lab technician will play along, show your child that the tourniquet really isn't a big deal. (Don't do this with the needle. It's best to hide the needle until it's time to draw the blood!) The lab technician needs to draw a small amount (about 3cc's) of blood—a process that takes a matter of minutes, if not seconds, but seems to take days.

The Endoscopy

If your child will be undergoing the endoscopy and biopsy, you have an ordeal ahead of you—for you more than for your child! Be sure to talk with her beforehand, and let her know that she is *so* lucky that she's having this test done, because the doctors might figure out what's making her feel icky, and she'll feel *so* much better soon.

The worst part for your child is the pre-surgical testing, which is usually done at the hospital the day before the surgery. They will do a "bleed" test that shows them how quickly your child's body stops its own bleeding. The nurse or assistant will prick your child's finger and then spend several minutes *squeezing* the blood out. Your child may feel she's going to bleed to death before it stops. There will also be a few other, less traumatic tests, and you will have a chance to talk with the anesthesiologist.

The night before the endoscopy, your child will not be able to eat or drink after a certain time. Usually this isn't a problem at night, but it can make the wait the next day miserable! Here you are, stressed and anxious, and your child is literally *screaming* for breakfast, a bottle, or just a small glass of water. It is so sad to deprive her, but it's extremely important. Don't give in, even to a small mint or piece of gum, as it could cause complications for the anesthesiologist.

The reason for forbidding food and drink is to minimize the volume of stomach contents so that regurgitation is less likely, and, if it does occur, aspiration will be less likely. But, according to anesthesiologist Richard Yoder, M.D., this has been a subject of many debates and varied management protocols in the anesthesia world, because when you don't feed the stomach for long periods of time, its contents become more acidic, and it's the acid that causes much of the aspiration damage. Regardless of the debate, always follow your anesthesiologist's advice.

Once you've gotten to the hospital, the fun begins. Your child gets to put on a strange-looking little "dress" that opens in the back and exposes her backside to everyone. At this point, ask a nurse or assistant if they have an extra anesthesia mask that your child can play with. Some hospitals will even spray the inside with a "bubble gum" or "grape" smell. Let your child choose her favorite smell, and then spend some time putting it on your face and hers. Explain that the doctors will need to hold this on her face for several minutes. Make sure she realizes she can breathe out of it, even though it may seem at first as though she can't.

Putting your child to sleep is a traumatic event. I wish I could have candy-coated that for you, but there's no way around it. Your doctor may not give you the option of being in the room, but I suggest you be very insistent upon it, unless you're particularly queasy. We held our son and put the mask on him. Yes, he struggled and it broke our hearts, but it was better that it was us than an anesthesiologist he didn't know. If you can handle it, I recommend you stay while your child goes under; then you may (definitely) want to leave.

You should stay in the hospital during the endoscopy, and even if you have to leave briefly, make sure you're there when your child wakes up. Some hospitals are good about calling you into the recovery room as your child starts to show signs of waking up. She will be disoriented at first, and often will have a sore throat from the endoscope. But she also gets yummy treats—usually a Popsicle. Make sure you tell her that it looks like the best Popsicle you've ever seen in your entire life, and talk about how much better she's going to start feeling. You can take your child home an hour or so after she wakes up.

For the first few days after the endoscopy, make sure you don't let your child eat ketchup or anything else red. You will need to observe her stools (or instruct caretakers to observe them) for a few days to make sure there are no internal perforations from the procedure, and a little bit of ketchup could just send you straight to the emergency room unnecessarily!

Self-Diagnosis: Trying Out the Gluten-Free Diet

Some parents choose to put their child on a gluten-free diet to judge for themselves whether there is any improvement. A trial of six weeks at a minimum is required to make any judgment about the success of the diet. Every child has a different reaction to the diet, and sometimes improvement takes time.

While signs of improvement *would*, in fact, indicate a high likelihood of celiac disease, it is important to proceed with formal testing and diagnosis. What if there are other conditions causing celiac-type symptoms, such as Crohn's disease or ulcerative colitis? What if your child's improvement upon introduction of a gluten-free diet is coincidental? It is important to know for sure. But remember, if you are going to proceed with formal testing, it is extremely important that your child be on a high-gluten-containing diet beforehand. Ask your doctor how long he recommends your child eat gluten prior to the testing.

Ongoing Testing

There are some tests that should be done periodically, even after your child has been diagnosed and is on a gluten-free diet.

The serum antibody test should be done every year, mostly to ensure that your child is, in fact, completely gluten-free. If there is some consumption, your child's antibody level may be elevated, and you can start searching for the culprit.

In addition, you should be aware that there are certain vitamin/mineral deficiency immunological disorders that are associated with celiac disease. People with celiac disease are more likely to have the following conditions than people without celiac disease, so you and your doctor should watch for symptoms:

- Dermatitis Herpetiformis (see Chapter Two)
- Diabetes (insulin-dependent)
- Thyroid disease
- Lupus
- Other autoimmune disorders

Who Else Should Be Tested?

Once you have a confirmed diagnosis of celiac disease in the family, every direct biological relative should be tested, even if they don't show any symptoms. As the previous chapter explains, celiac disease is a genetic disorder, and that means that one or both of the parents is at least a carrier of the gene, if not an actual celiac. A carrier is someone who passes a particular gene on to his or her child, but doesn't exhibit symptoms.

Recent research indicates that as many as 10 to 30 percent of first-degree relatives of people diagnosed with celiac disease have either symptomatic or asymptomatic celiac disease. There is a 30-to-40-times increased risk of having celiac disease compared with those who have no family history of celiac disease.* It doesn't matter which relatives are tested first; the gene could be on both sides of the family, so everyone should be included in the testing round-up. Be pre-

---

* Karoly Horvath, M.D., as written in *Gluten-Free Living Magazine,* January/February 1999.

pared, because most likely, you *will* get resistance, if not flat-out refusals, when you suggest that your relatives be tested. It might be a good idea to share with them the upcoming section on "The Consequences of Misdiagnosis."

Getting Siblings Tested

There is about a 30 percent chance that brothers and sisters will have the condition, so it is especially important to have them tested. It doesn't matter how old the siblings are, as long as they're eating a gluten-containing diet.

If you have a baby in addition to a child who has been diagnosed with celiac disease, it is a good idea to keep the baby gluten-free for the first year of her life. The question of whether or not nursing mothers can pass gluten through their breast milk has been debated for years. Recent studies seem to indicate that gluten is not, in fact, passed from a nursing mother to her baby. However, if there is reason to suspect that your baby might have celiac disease (because it runs in the family), it would be safest for the nursing mother to avoid gluten until the baby has been weaned. You should also know that many formulas are gluten-free, including the soy-based, lactose-free varieties (be sure to check with the manufacturer to be sure).

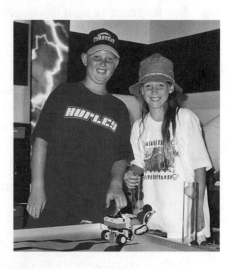

Once your baby is a year old, slowly and selectively begin to add gluten to the diet, watching for any of the "classic" symptoms. (See Chapter Two for a list of these symptoms.) Of course, if there are any indications of gastrointestinal distress or abnormalities, see your pediatrician and ask for a referral to a pediatric gastroenterologist. If, however, your child has been eased onto a completely "normal" (gluten-containing) diet with no symptoms whatsoever, you can assume that it is *likely* (but not for sure) that she does not have celiac disease. Even so, it is a good idea to have a serum antibody test done by age three or so, even if symptoms are not apparent.

Other People Who Should Be Tested

People with Conditions That Carry a Higher Risk of Celiac Disease

Even if they do not have any relatives diagnosed with celiac disease, people with the following conditions should be tested for celiac disease. This is true even if they exhibit none of the "classic" gastrointestinal symptoms.

- Type 1 diabetes mellitus
- Any other autoimmune disorder
- Down syndrome

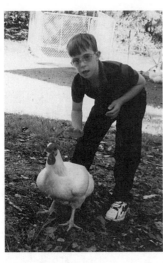

- Cystic fibrosis
- Chronic active hepatitis
- Scleroderma
- Sjogren syndrome
- Raynaud syndrome
- Addison's disease
- Myasthenia gravis
- Rheumatoid arthritis
- Epilepsy or cerebral calcifications

The reason people with the above conditions should be tested for celiac disease is that they are more likely to have celiac disease than other people. These conditions do not necessarily *cause* celiac disease, but for some reason the conditions are associated with an increased risk of having celiac disease. For example, studies of people with Down syndrome have found incidences of celiac disease ranging between 5 and 16 percent.

People with Conditions That Can Be Caused by Celiac Disease

People with the following conditions should also be tested for celiac disease. In these cases, celiac disease itself can be what causes the conditions:

- Selective IgA deficiency
- Unexplained anemia
- Deficiency in folic acid and other vitamins/minerals/nutrients
- Infertility
- Osteoporosis
- Growth retardation, short stature, failure to thrive
- Delayed puberty in children and adolescents

People with Conditions That May Be Associated with Celiac Disease

It has been hypothesized that the disorders listed below *may* be associated with an increased incidence of celiac disease, but no direct links to celiac disease have been proven.

- Autism
- Attention-deficit/hyperactivity disorder (ADHD)
- Multiple sclerosis (MS)
- Lactose intolerance
- Fibromyalgia
- ITP (Immune Thrombocytopenic Purpura)

Some people with these conditions may improve when put on a strict gluten-free diet, while others show no change. Because these underlying conditions are serious in nature, you should always advise your pediatrician of your intent to experiment with the gluten-free diet. In addition to needing to monitor your child's health, your doctor may have valuable input that would help you measure the results of the diet more effectively, too.

Remember that if you plan to test for the presence of anti-gluten antibodies, your child must be eating gluten. So, if you think you'll want the testing done and are interested in trying the diet, get the antibody test done *before* eliminating gluten from your child's diet.

The Consequences of Misdiagnosis

Chapter Two gave a laundry list of complications that may develop when someone with celiac disease continues to consume gluten. To help you understand why putting your child on a gluten-free diet is essential, as well as to convince any doubting relatives that getting themselves tested for celiac disease is a wise move, this section examines a few of the more common complications in detail.

Lactose Intolerance

Before diagnosis, many people with celiac disease suffer from some degree of lactose intolerance, which is an inability to tolerate lactose, (a sugar found in dairy products). People with lactose intolerance may feel symptoms of gas, bloating, cramping, or diarrhea whenever they eat dairy products.

The reason people with celiac disease develop lactose intolerance is because the tips of the villi typically produce *lactase*—an enzyme that helps in digesting the lactose in dairy products. If the villi are damaged by exposure to gluten, the production of lactase may sometimes be interrupted, resulting in a lactose "intolerance."

Once someone with celiac disease starts adhering to a strict gluten-free diet, the small intestine repairs itself, and healthy villi are again usually able to produce lactase. Usually the lactose intolerance then disappears. (Of course, some people will be lactose intolerant regardless of the celiac condition.) Some physicians suggest keeping your child off of lactose for a few months after beginning the gluten-free diet. Not only will this give your child's gut plenty of time to become healthy again, but if the symptoms did not disappear and lactose was still part of the diet, you would be unsure about whether the symptoms were caused by the lactose, the gluten, or both. See Chapter Twenty-Three for more information about lactose intolerance.

Effects on Bones

People with celiac disease who continue to eat gluten can suffer from bone loss (osteoporosis), or, in children, slowed or stunted growth. The reason for this is a calcium deficiency. Remember that the damage done by gluten occurs at the beginning of the small intestine. This is the same area where calcium is absorbed. Another reason for calcium deficiency is that when people with celiac disease continue to eat gluten, they do not absorb fat-soluble vitamins, including vitamin D, which plays a critical role in the body's processing of calcium.

Calcium absorption is critical in the formation of children's bones, as well as for women who are approaching menopause or are post-menopausal and are at risk for osteoporosis.

Many doctors recommend that people with celiac disease get a bone density test to determine the degree of bone loss, if any. Some also recommend giving the child calcium supplements, at least in the initial stages of introducing a gluten-free diet.

The good news is that just as the body is able to repair the small intestine once it is on a strict gluten-free diet, bone density in children returns to normal as well. Adults with celiac disease who already have osteoporosis may be able to prevent further effects on their bones by adopting a gluten-free diet, but their bones will not return to normal. (This is just one important reason to advocate the earliest possible diagnosis of celiac disease: after years of eating a gluten-containing diet, people with celiac disease can develop irreversible bone loss.)

Infertility and Complications of Pregnancy

This book is intended to focus on children with celiac disease, and they're obviously not getting pregnant. But this is an important issue to address, because many of the family members (mothers, sisters, aunts) of celiac kids may be at risk for reproductive problems.

Women with unrecognized celiac disease who want to get pregnant face two risks associated with their condition: a higher chance of infertility, and a higher risk of having a baby with a birth defect. Research has shown that men may also have infertility problems as a result of celiac disease.

For women who have celiac disease but don't know it, the most likely explanation for increased risk of birth defects is that they are eating gluten, suffering (maybe without even knowing it) from malabsorption, and are deficient in important nutrients. They assume that because they're eating a healthy diet, they are getting the important nutrients. In fact, they can be severely deficient, especially in folic acid and iron.

Folic acid plays a critical role in the development of a fetus, especially at the very beginning of the pregnancy, when a woman may not even know she is pregnant. A deficiency in folic acid is one of the main factors in the development of neural tube defects such as anencephaly (absence of a brain) and spina bifida.

In fact, in March 2000, a study conducted in Italy concluded that pregnant women should routinely be tested for celiac disease*. The researchers pointed

---

* *Gut* 2000; 46: 332-335.

out that celiac disease is far more common than most of the diseases for which pregnant women are routinely screened.

"Up to 50% of women with untreated coeliac disease experience miscarriage or an unfavourable outcome of pregnancy. In most cases, after 6-12 months of a gluten-free diet, no excess of unfavourable outcome of pregnancy is observed."

It is important to note that women with celiac disease who are gluten-free face no additional risks in pregnancy due to celiac disease. Nutritional supplements and specific prenatal vitamins are always recommended, regardless of whether or not celiac disease is present.

Research: What the Future Holds for People with Celiac Disease

For decades, celiac disease research was limited in the United States, probably because it wasn't considered a "dire" condition. After all, there is no medication required, no surgery, and a healthy prognosis with "simply" a dietary modification. Today, however, there is quite a bit of research activity here in the United States as well as in Europe and elsewhere.

In fact, in the last few years, there has been a much greater emphasis on researching the disease. The ultimate goal, of course, is to find some sort of a "cure," but scientists are also looking at ways to make the body able to "tolerate" foods that normally would cause a reaction in people with celiac disease. One of the newest findings, announced by British researchers in early 2000, is that it might be possible to genetically engineer wheat so as to be nontoxic to people with celiac disease. Or, it might be possible to make *peptides,* or short proteins, that could switch off the immune response in people with celiac disease.

Zonulin

One of the newest discoveries in celiac disease was made early in 2000 by University of Maryland researchers, who found that a protein called zonulin reaches higher levels in patients with celiac disease.

Zonulin acts like a "gatekeeper" for the body's tissues. It opens the spaces between the cells, allowing some substances to pass through, while preventing harmful bacteria and toxins from entering.

People with celiac disease have higher levels of zonulin, which, in essence, leaves the gates "stuck open," allowing gluten and other harmful substances to pass through.

In the medical journal *Lancet,* Alessio Fasano, M.D., explained, "We could never understand how a big protein like gluten was getting through the immune system." But in people with celiac disease, who are now known to have higher levels of zonulin, the "gates" stay open. "The consequence," said Fasano, "is that everything in the intestine can get into the (immune system), including large molecules like gluten."

As a consequence of this discovery, researchers, including Fasano, are working on a compound that prevents zonulin from binding to key receptors in the intestine. "If our hypothesis is correct," Fasano predicted," we will have the potential to protect people from serious diseases," including celiac disease and a variety of other autoimmune diseases.

The Prognosis

Consider your child blessed if she is diagnosed with celiac disease. Although she will never outgrow celiac disease, no medications or surgical procedures are required to ensure her a lifetime of happiness and good health. Internally, her small intestine will return to a perfectly "normal" state, and there will be no traces of the havoc that gluten wreaked. Keeping your child on a strict gluten-free diet is all it takes. Okay, the diet isn't exactly a piece of gluten-free cake, but that's what this book is for. Remember, *deal with it—don't dwell on it!*

23 Nutrition Basics

Nancy Patin Falini, M.A., R.D.

Perhaps you are wondering why there is such a long chapter on the nutritional needs of children with celiac disease if "all" you have to do is cut out gluten from your child's diet. True, the nutritional needs of children with celiac disease are the same as other children's when their celiac disease is controlled. But figuring out how to give your child a balanced diet when so many foods are forbidden can be difficult, at least in the beginning. In addition, before your child's celiac disease is controlled, he can have nutritional deficiencies. And, as with any children, you may encounter special nutritional issues, such as a child who wants to become a vegetarian, or one who goes on food jags, or one who needs additional calories.

This chapter is meant to answer your questions about all of these issues, and to let you know when or if you need to handle them differently for your child with celiac disease.

The Food Guide Pyramid

It is important for all families—with and without children with celiac disease—to learn to use the Food Guide Pyramid to their nutritional advantage. The Food Guide Pyramid (shown below) has replaced the Four Food Groups you may have learned about in school. It is a visual presentation of how to classify foods based on similar nutrient content and how much to consume from each food group daily. Ultimately, its use should result in a nutritious, well-balanced diet with appropriate servings based on five food groups.

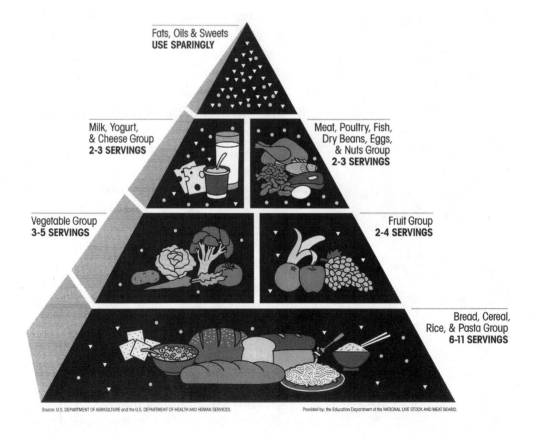

Fats, Oils & Sweets
USE SPARINGLY

Milk, Yogurt,
& Cheese Group
2-3 SERVINGS

Meat, Poultry, Fish,
Dry Beans, Eggs,
& Nuts Group
2-3 SERVINGS

Vegetable Group
3-5 SERVINGS

Fruit Group
2-4 SERVINGS

Bread, Cereal,
Rice, & Pasta Group
6-11 SERVINGS

Source: U.S. DEPARTMENT OF AGRICULTURE and the U.S. DEPARTMENT OF HEALTH AND HUMAN SERVICES.   Provided by: the Education Department of the NATIONAL LIVE STOCK AND MEAT BOARD.

Using the Food Guide Pyramid to help plan meals and snacks and direct your food shopping is a practical way to make the pyramid work for you. Keep in mind that the pyramid serves as a general guide for people aged two to seventy. (There is a modified pyramid for adults after age seventy.) A new diagnosis of celiac disease may, however, warrant the need to modify the principals of the Food Guide Pyramid. For example, your child might benefit from eating more high protein foods than generally recommended during his initial recovery from celiac disease.

When applying the principles of the Food Guide Pyramid, the lower on the pyramid a food is, the better. In other words, it's best to base your diet on the food groups that are represented at the base of the pyramid rather than those closer to, or at, the top. As you can see in the Food Guide Pyramid above, plant foods (which are high in carbohydrates) are at the base, while animal foods (which are high in protein and provide varying levels of fat and cholesterol) are at the higher level. Oils/fats (which are pure sources of fat), such as cooking oil, butter, and sweets (which are high in carbohydrate and generally high in fat) are at the top. Oils/fats and sweets are not to be eliminated, but should be used moderately to add enjoyment to eating and complement food flavor. Oils/fats also have nutritional value.

Following the Food Guide Pyramid will help you and your family eat adequate amounts of the six types of nutrients: carbohydrate, protein, fat, vitamins, minerals, and water.

Carbohydrate, protein, and fat are *macronutrients*. These all provide energy in the form of calories. The primary function of protein is to promote growth and tissue production, including skin, hair, and muscle. When too much protein is consumed, it is used as energy or stored as calories.

Vitamins and minerals are *micronutrients*. They do not supply calories. They enable the body to metabolize the macronutrients. They help to regulate necessary bodily processes that are required for good health, as well as prevent disease.

Water, the sixth nutrient, is in a class of its own. Water is the medium in which the other nutrients function. It also helps regulate body temperature and maintain regularity of bowel movements.

The Five Food Groups

Below is an explanation of each of the five food groups with a range of recommended numbers of servings and serving sizes. These servings are to be spread out among meals and snacks throughout each day. Please note that for children ages two to three, all of the serving sizes may be reduced to approximately two-thirds the standard serving size, with the exception of the Milk, Yogurt, & Cheese Group. The serving size for this food group is the same as for children four years and older.

The Food Guide Pyramid is not designed to meet the specific needs of infants and children under two. Your pediatrician or local registered dietitian can provide guidelines for your infant or child this age.

Bread, Cereal, Rice, and Pasta Group (also referred to as the Bread and Cereal Group)

- Number of servings each day: 6-11
- Examples of serving sizes for ages four and older: 1 slice bread; ½ cup cooked cereal, rice, pasta; 1 ounce dry cereal; 5-6 medium crackers; or 1 medium size muffin.

Some children with celiac disease eat too few breads and cereals, especially if a limited variety is offered to them. Instead, they may fill up on cookies, cakes, and candy to replace the calories (energy) normally obtained from this food group. Needless to say, this is a situation that parents should try to avoid!

Whenever possible, provide these foods to your child with celiac disease in the form of unrefined whole grains and enriched grains, such as:

- flaxseed meal/milled flaxseed,
- brown rice and its flour,
- rice bran and rice polish,
- enriched white rice,
- enriched rice baby cereal and cream of rice,
- stone ground whole kernel corn tortillas,
- enriched cornmeal and corn flour.

Also take advantage of flours made from beans—such as chickpea and fava bean flour—and nut flours, such as almond flour. (Full fat rather than partially defatted nut flours are more nutritious.) All of these are more nutritious than the standard gluten-free unenriched rice flour that is so commonly used in gluten-free bread and cereal products.

Foods from this group are important because they provide complex carbohydrates (which includes fiber); some B vitamins, such as thiamin; and minerals, such as iron and zinc. Phytochemicals are also provided. These are naturally occurring substances in plant foods that appear to play a role in helping to ward off the development of some chronic diseases.

Fruit and Vegetable Groups

Fruits:

- Number of servings each day: 2-4
- Examples of serving sizes for ages four and older: 1 piece of fruit or melon wedge; ½ cup chopped or canned fruit; ¾ cup fruit juice; or ¼ cup dried fruit.

Vegetables:

- Number of servings each day: 3-5
- Examples of serving sizes for ages four and older: 1 cup raw, leafy vegetables; ½ cup chopped, raw, or cooked vegetables; ½ cup potato salad; or ¾ cup vegetable juice.

Because fruits and vegetables are high in fiber, a child who is recovering from diarrhea and/or bloating and gas may need to avoid eating them raw until substantial healing has begun. (See the section on "Carbohydrates," below.) Eating soft, peeled, and cooked fruits and vegetables will help increase nutrient absorption while preventing further aggravation of celiac gastrointestinal symptoms. Children under the age of two, with or without celiac disease, should also make a gradual transition from soft or cooked fruits and vegetables to raw ones.

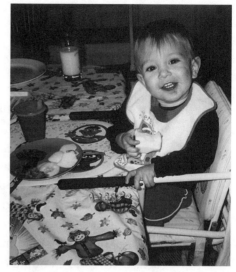

If your child does not care for fresh vegetables, don't worry! Cooked frozen vegetables are not inferior to fresh vegetables. Frozen vegetables can be just as nutritious, if not more so. One reason is that as fresh vegetables sit in your refrigerator, over time they lose their nutrient content. If this is the norm in your home, remember to eat fresh veggies up quickly or purchase frozen vegetables. This applies to fresh fruit as well. Once it enters your home, it should be devoured promptly.

Both of these food groups can supply a variety of minerals and vitamins, such as vitamin A (in the form of carotene) and vitamin C—both of which aid in preventing infection and are antioxidants. Antioxidants provide protection against chronic disease, such as malignancy and heart disease.

Everyone in your family should consume at least one or two good sources of vitamin A (carotene) daily from either the fruit or vegetable food group. Good sources of vitamin A include:

- apricots,
- peaches,
- cantaloupe,
- carrots,
- sweet potatoes,
- yams,
- dark green, leafy vegetables such as broccoli, kale, collard greens.

Also consume a minimum of one good vitamin C source daily, such as:

- citrus fruit,
- kiwi,
- strawberries,
- honeydew,
- vitamin C enriched fruit juice,
- tomatoes,

- Brussels sprouts,
- broccoli,
- spinach,
- white potatoes.

When these key vitamins are sufficient in the diet, it is believed that other vital nutrients are, as well.

Meat, Poultry, Fish, Dry Beans, Eggs, and Nuts Group (also referred to as the Meat Group)

- Number of servings each day: 2-3
- Examples of serving sizes for ages four and older: 1 serving equals 2-3 ounces of cooked lean meat, poultry, or fish (the size of a deck of cards is a visual example of a 3-ounce serving). Note: ½ cup cooked dried beans, peas, or lentils, 4 ounces of tofu, 1 whole egg, 2 tablespoons of nut or seed butters, ⅓ cup nuts, or ¼ to ½ cup seeds count as 1 ounce of meat, poultry, or fish.

Some children with celiac disease, especially adolescents, may consume too much meat. This can result in an excessive intake of protein, as well as fat and cholesterol.

As you can see, this group doesn't just include meat. Legumes (dried beans and peas, lentils, and peanuts), nuts (tree nuts), and seeds are also classified here. So, three 3-ounce servings from this group can be met a variety of ways. For example, 1 egg, 3 ounces of sliced turkey, 2 tablespoons of peanut butter, 1 cup of beans, and 2 ounces of ground beef/pork (over the course of a day) provide the equivalent of 9 ounces from this particular food group. (Of course, depending on your child's age and individual needs, he may need less than 9 ounces from this food group.)

To get more nutrition for your money *and* reduce the risk of encountering hidden gluten, serve lean, fresh meat and poultry frequently and processed meats such as hot dogs less often. Whole nuts and seeds should not be given until your child is at least two years of age and has all his teeth. Also use discretion when serving nut and seed butters to younger children. Butters such as almond butter and sunflower butter can be thick and dry and may be difficult to swallow for some children.

Foods in this group supply protein, varying levels of fat, iron, and B vitamins. In addition, the foods specifically from animals supply cholesterol, vitamin B12, zinc, selenium, and chromium. Dried beans, peas, and lentils provide folate and phytochemicals and some calcium. Soybeans have been identified as a *prebiotic*. Because of their unique carbohydrate composition, they have been shown to stimulate the growth of healthy intestinal bacteria*. This can help prevent bacte-

---

* Nadeau, D. "Oligosaccharides Play Important Health Role." *The Soy Connection.* Summer 1999; 7.

rial overgrowth (excess production of bacteria in the small intestine), which can occur in some medical conditions, including celiac disease. Nuts and seeds contain vitamin E, as well as copper, magnesium, fiber, and phytochemicals.

Milk, Yogurt, and Cheese Group (also referred to as the Dairy Group)
- Number of servings each day: 2-3
- Examples of serving sizes for ages two and older: 1 cup milk, yogurt, or pudding; 1½ ounces hard, natural cheese like cheddar; 2 ounces processed cheese like American; 2 cups cottage cheese; or 1½ cups ice cream.

Until age two, children should consume whole milk and whole milk dairy products. After this age, they can switch to lower fat versions. Whenever possible, choose vitamin D-fortified dairy products, such as milk, yogurt, and cottage cheese.

This food group is rich in various bone- and teeth-building nutrients, including calcium, vitamin D (when fortified with it), and phosphorus, as well as relatively smaller amounts of vitamin K. B vitamins, such as riboflavin, are also provided.

If your child develops gas, diarrhea, or other uncomfortable symptoms after consuming dairy products, see the section on "Disaccharide Intolerance" below.

Nutrient Imbalances and Deficiencies Related to Celiac Disease

Celiac disease primarily affects the upper part of the small intestine (duodenum). This is where the gluten initially enters the intestinal tract from the stomach. The damage can be mild to severe and can eventually progress to the middle part of the small intestine (jejunum) and to the lower part of the small intestine (ileum). (See the illustration on page 3.)

In active celiac disease, the absorption of all nutrients may potentially be affected. The extent of intestinal damage and the length of time between the onset of the disease and diagnosis generally determines which nutrients are malabsorbed. Generally, the more extensive the damage, the greater the malabsorption of nutrients. In some people, however, the areas that are not damaged compensate and absorb nutrients that would otherwise be malabsorbed, thereby preventing nutrient imbalances and deficiencies.

One of the advantages of being diagnosed with celiac disease during childhood is that the body is so resilient. Once gluten is removed, symptoms start to resolve within a few days. Within six to twelve months, the small intestine completely heals.

The following information will help familiarize you with the nutrients that tend to be malabsorbed, and the signs that can identify their imbalances or deficiencies. To help correct these conditions, good food sources of these nutrients are listed.

Carbohydrates

Especially when the jejunum is damaged, all forms of carbohydrates may be malabsorbed, from cellulose and starch to disaccharides. Disaccharide intolerance is discussed in greater detail later in this chapter.

Signs of Imbalances or Deficiencies: Growth retardation, weight loss, fatigue, concentration problems, and gastrointestinal symptoms, as explained in the Disaccharide Intolerance section.

Good Food Sources: The three lower food groups on the Food Guide Pyramid are good sources of carbohydrates, as well as dried beans, peas, lentils, and some dairy products. If your child is experiencing diarrhea, it may be better for him to consume low fiber carbohydrates rather than higher fiber ones. This would include providing cooked vegetables over raw vegetables and salads; fruit without the skin and seeds; canned fruit; and refined enriched bread and cereal products. Once nutrient absorption begins to improve, your child can slowly integrate higher fiber foods into his diet, while being sure to drink adequate fluid.

Protein

Protein is made up of amino acids (the building blocks of protein). Malabsorption of protein can occur if there is damage to your child's duodenum and jejunum.

Signs of Imbalances or Deficiencies: Muscle wasting, fluid accumulation (edema) especially in ankles and feet, growth retardation, and weight loss.

Good Food Sources: Excellent sources of protein are from animal foods in the dairy and meat groups. Bread and cereal products, legumes, nuts, and seeds supply smaller amounts of protein. Commercially designed liquid supplemental drinks, such as Kindercal, Pediasure, and Ensure, are good protein sources.

Fat

Fat malabsorption can occur when the jejunum is damaged. In addition, pancreatic insufficiency, which can result from the intestinal damage caused by celiac disease, can contribute to fat malabsorption.

Signs of Imbalances or Deficiencies: Weight and growth can be altered. Bowel movements characteristic of *steatorrhea* may appear. These are bulky, pale, greasy bowel movements that can emit a rancid odor. Over time, an essential fatty acid deficiency may develop, resulting in symptoms such as eczema/dermatitis or *follicular hyperkeratosis,* a condition in which the hair follicles, primarily on the arms, are prominent.

Good Food Sources: Oils and fats, cooking oils, margarine, butter, shortening, olives, nuts, seeds. Good sources specifically of essential fatty acids are oils, as well as soft, pourable spreads from any of these sources: flaxseed, canola, safflower, soybean, corn, peanut, cottonseed, sesame, sunflower, or walnut*. Whole walnuts, soy nuts, sunflower seeds, peanuts, and flaxseeds also supply essential fatty acids. Fish, such as salmon and white tuna, soy flour, and soy beverages do too.

When fat malabsorption is severe enough, the use of M.C.T. oil (medium chain triglycerides) under the supervision of a physician may be required. Since medium chain triglycerides are more easily absorbed, M.C.T. oil may be used solely as fat calories or replace some of the fat calories (from cooking oil, margarine, butter) in the diet until adequate fat absorption returns. M.C.T. oil does not contain essential fatty acids. In my experience, M.C.T. oil is rarely necessary as long as the child avoids fatty and fried foods, consumes a diet moderate in fat, and totally eliminates gluten. Again, because children are so resilient, steatorrhea usually improves within a few days of starting a gluten-free diet.

Fat Soluble Vitamins (Vitamins A, D, E, K)

Malabsorption of vitamins A, D, E, and K can occur when the duodenum is damaged. In addition, the malabsorption of these vitamins is worsened when there are difficulties absorbing fat. This is because fat ordinarily acts as a carrier and enables vitamins A, D, E, and K to be absorbed. If your child's fat absorption is seriously impaired, he may need to take vitamin supplements of *water miscible fat soluble vitamins* (fat soluble vitamins not requiring fat for absorption) until his absorption improves.

Signs of Imbalances or Deficiencies: Steatorrhea can indicate the malabsorption of all of the fat soluble vitamins and over time can contribute to deficiencies of these vitamins. Signs of specific vitamin deficiencies include:

- *Vitamin A/Carotene* (plant source of vitamin A): Follicular hyperkeratosis, eyes becoming dry and hard, night blindness.
- *Vitamin D:* Bone disease, including osteomalacia or rickets, which rarely occurs in the U.S.A.; osteoporosis (loss of bone mass); and muscle twitching (*tetany*).
- *Vitamin E:* Neurological abnormalities, such as impaired reflexes.
- *Vitamin K:* Prolonged bleeding, spontaneous nose bleeds, bruising.

Good Food Sources:
- *Vitamin A/Carotene:* Vitamin A-fortified milk; eggs; liver; dark green, deep orange, and yellow vegetables and fruit, such as spinach, carrots, yams, and various types of squash, cantaloupe, apricots.

---

* "Fishing for Omega-3s." *Food & Fitness Advisor.* April 1999.

- *Vitamin D:* Vitamin D-fortified dairy products and milk alternatives, such as rice, soy, and almond beverages; organ meats; egg yolks; fatty fish such as salmon and sardines. Also, exposing the skin, including at least the hands and face, to sunlight for a minimum of fifteen minutes, three times a week over the majority of each year, generally allows for the production of vitamin D in the skin.
- *Vitamin E:* Vegetable oils, margarine, nuts, and seeds.
- *Vitamin K:* Dark green, leafy vegetables, such as spinach, broccoli, and kale are good sources. Dairy foods and eggs contain some. The healthy intestine makes vitamin K by the presence of bacteria.

Calcium

Regardless of the level of intestinal damage, malabsorption of this mineral seems to occur in all degrees of celiac disease.

Signs of Imbalances or Deficiencies: As with vitamin D deficiency, osteomalacia, rickets, and osteoporosis. Also retarded bone age, back and leg pains, heart palpitations, and muscle twitching. The presence of steatorrhea suggests that calcium is likely being malabsorbed. This is because malabsorbed fat attaches to calcium and prevents its absorption.

Good Food Sources: Dairy foods tend to be excellent sources. Also calcium-fortified orange juice; rice, soy, almond beverages; and tofu processed with calcium. Dried beans, peas, and lentils provide lower amounts. See the section on Disaccharide Intolerance for more sources.

Magnesium

This is another mineral that is often malabsorbed by people with active celiac disease. It works in harmony with calcium, both in the blood and the bones[*].

Signs of Imbalances or Deficiencies: Osteoporosis, muscle twitching and cramping, insomnia, irritability, depression, fatigue, weakness.

Good Food Sources: Legumes, tofu, nuts, such as almonds and hazelnuts, brown rice, and dark green, leafy vegetables such as spinach are some good sources.

Zinc

There is evidence that the level of this mineral is affected in active celiac disease and is more likely to be deficient when persistent diarrhea exists. To further complicate matters, a national survey recently revealed that children ages one to six and adolescents (with or without celiac disease) are at risk for consuming less than ideal amounts of zinc.

---

* Rude, R., and M. Olerich. "Magnesium Deficiency: Possible Role in Osteoporosis Associated with Gluten-Sensitive Enteropathy." *Osteoporosis International* 1996; 6:453-461.

Signs of Imbalances or Deficiencies: Loss of taste and appetite (anorexia), delayed healing, increased susceptibility to infection, retarded growth, hair loss.

Good Food Sources: Meat, liver, and seafood are the best sources, while legumes, soybeans, and whole grains are good sources.

Iron

Iron is frequently malabsorbed by people with active celiac disease. This is not necessarily the sole cause of iron deficiency, however. Iron lost through bleeding from the damaged intestine may also contribute.

Signs of Imbalances or Deficiencies: Iron deficiency anemia (fewer than normal red blood cells) and microcytic anemia (abnormally small red blood cells). Also, one study found that children who have celiac disease and develop iron deficiency anemia may also develop *pica*. Pica is compulsive eating of non-food items, such as dirt and sand, and is associated with iron deficiency. Fatigue, weakness, retarded growth, and pale skin may also result from anemia.

Good Food Sources: There are two types of iron present in food: heme iron (from animal tissue) and non-heme iron (from plant foods). Heme iron is better absorbed and is contained in meat, poultry, seafood, and organ meats. Non-heme sources include legumes, nuts, seeds, whole grains, enriched bread and cereal products, and dark green, leafy vegetables. To improve absorption of non-heme iron, your child should simultaneously consume a good source of vitamin C. This can include citrus fruit, berries, dark, leafy green vegetables, or cruciferous vegetables (broccoli, cauliflower, cabbage). Iron-fortified infant formula is another source of iron and may be used to replace milk even after infancy.

Folate/Folic Acid

The malabsorption of this B vitamin is common in people with active celiac disease. Folic acid is the manmade form of folate, and is better absorbed than the natural form. Folic acid is used in vitamin supplements and in the fortification of foods.

Signs of Imbalances or Deficiencies: Macrocytic anemia (enlarged red blood cells), smooth tongue (glossitis), mental confusion. Seizures associated with celiac disease can occur but do not appear to be common. They are thought to be caused by calcium deposits in the brain from folate deficiency.

Good Food Sources: Vegetables and fruits, such as dark green, leafy vegetables, oranges, strawberries, legumes, and folic acid-fortified bread and cereal products, such as cornmeal, grits, and rice.

Vitamin B12 (Cobalamin)

An important role of this B vitamin is to work with folic acid to make red blood cells. Malabsorption of vitamin B12 is rarely an issue for children with celiac disease*, but it may occur in adolescents. This vitamin is not absorbed until it reaches the ileum—the end of the small intestine—so celiac damage must spread to this area of the intestine for absorption to be affected. Children may also be protected from deficiencies because they may have accumulated stores of vitamin B12 in their liver before birth. If malabsorption does occur, bacterial overgrowth in the intestine may be responsible.

Signs of Imbalances or Deficiencies: Deficiencies are rare in infants and children, but may occur in adolescents. A deficiency state results in megaloblastic anemia (enlarged and irregular red blood cells) and pernicious anemia, which can produce symptoms such as loss of balance and numbness and tingling in fingers and toes. Also, fatigue, smooth tongue, and skin sensitivity can occur.

Good Food Sources: All animal foods: meat, poultry, seafood, organ meats, eggs, and dairy foods.

Potassium, Sodium, Chloride (Electrolytes)

These are very important minerals that work together to regulate fluid balance and transmit nerve impulses. Potassium and sodium also affect muscle function. These minerals can become imbalanced or deficient when the jejunum is damaged, or if your child experiences chronic diarrhea or vomiting. Damage in the duodenum can also affect chloride absorption.

Signs of Imbalances or Deficiencies: These are somewhat similar for all three minerals. They include, but are not limited to, nausea, muscle cramps, weakness, fatigue, chronic diarrhea, and vomiting. *Celiac crisis,* a shock-like state, is a condition in which an infant or very young child experiences a sudden onset of watery diarrhea and vomiting. This condition can be a result of depleted electrolytes.

Good Food Sources: For potassium, these include fruits and vegetables, such as bananas, apricots, cantaloupe, grapefruit, oranges, kiwi, potatoes, and tomatoes, as well as dairy products and fresh meat, poultry, and seafood. Both sodium and chloride are found in table salt (sodium chloride) and in processed foods containing table salt. Sodium is also present naturally in a variety of foods, such as certain types of vegetables.

Disaccharide Intolerance (Including Lactose Intolerance)

As discussed above, carbohydrate malabsorption does occur in celiac disease. The malabsorption can be significant enough to involve even small mol-

---

* Green, P., and F. Byfield. "The Diagnosis of Celiac Disease 1998." *Clinical Perspectives in Gastroenterology* 1998; 1:133-139.

ecules of carbohydrate. This can lead to an *intolerance* of (or inability to process) foods containing carbohydrates.

Ordinarily, the small molecules of carbohydrates, also known as *disaccharides,* are digested by *disaccharidases*—enzymes released from the villi. An intolerance to any one or all of the disaccharides can occur if celiac disease damages the villi. *Lactase* is the first disaccharidase deficiency to occur and the last to become normal. Lactase is the enzyme that digests lactose, or milk sugar. There may also be deficiencies in the disaccharidases *sucrase,* the enzyme that digests sucrose (white sugar, brown sugar, and syrups), and *maltase,* the enzyme that digests maltose, a nearly completely digested version of starch.

When damaged villi no longer produce the enzymes needed to digest carbohydrates, disaccharides pass into the small intestine undigested. When the undigested disaccharides enter the small intestine, they attract water, which produces diarrhea. As they make their way through the large intestine/colon, they are fermented to acids and gases by naturally occurring intestinal bacteria. This results in flatulence, bloating, or abdominal distension. Cramps and nausea also may occur. These symptoms usually show up within thirty minutes to two hours after consuming the disaccharide*.

Keep in mind that a disaccharidase deficiency does not damage the intestine like gluten does. It is a secondary result of gluten damage. Incidentally, persistent diarrhea (regardless of the cause) damages the villi, thus contributing to malabsorption.

Lactose Intolerance

Not surprisingly, most people newly diagnosed with celiac disease have some degree of lactose intolerance. Some, however, do not seem to have symptoms, probably because their lactose consumption does not exceed their individual level of tolerance. Most of those who do have symptoms will get over their lactose intolerance after they have been on a gluten-free diet long enough for their intestines to heal substantially or completely. Generally speaking, the level of mucosal damage and the rate of healing determine how long it takes for the lactose intolerance to resolve.

Although there are formal tests for lactose intolerance, many physicians base a diagnosis on the presence of the characteristic symptoms associated with dairy product consumption. Some, however, simultaneously evaluate for lactase deficiency while they are obtaining a biopsy to test for celiac disease.

The amount of lactose your child will need to eliminate depends on the degree of his lactase deficiency. You will also learn through trial and error how much, if any lactose, your child can tolerate. Babies and young children up until

---

* National Digestive Diseases Information Clearinghouse. "Lactose Intolerance Fact Sheet." April 1994.

the age of two or so should completely eliminate all forms of lactose until the intolerance is resolved. This is also true of anyone who has a severe intolerance. For many children, however, just limiting the types and/or amounts of dairy products is all that is necessary. Because dairy products are so nutritious, they should be incorporated into your child's diet as tolerated.

If your child has a lactose intolerance, you need to be aware that lactose may be an ingredient in other foods besides dairy products. These may include whey, curds, milk byproducts, dry milk solids, cream, and nonfat dry milk powder. Lactose may also be used as an inactive ingredient in vitamin and mineral supplements and medications.

If your child has a temporary or permanent lactose intolerance, here are some products and strategies that may help him get the calcium, as well as other nutrients, he needs. These are to be used based on individual needs and tolerance.

Calcium-Rich and Lactose-Free and Reduced Products:

- Lactose-free infant formulas, such as those that are soy based or hydrolyzed
- Liquid supplemental drinks, such as Kindercal, Boost (made by Mead Johnson), Pediasure, Osmolite, and Ensure (made by Ross Medical Nutritional Line)
- Commercial lactose-reduced or lactose-free milk
- Commercial lactase enzyme droplets to add to milk; caplets or tablets to consume with lactose-containing products
- Vance's Non Dairy Beverage Mix
- Calcium-, and, ideally, vitamin D-fortified, rice, soy, and almond beverages
- Calcium-fortified orange juice

Other Nondairy Sources of Calcium:

- Dried beans, peas, and lentils, such as kidney, navy, red, or black beans and chick peas/garbanzo beans
- Dark green, leafy vegetables, such as broccoli and Chinese cabbage (bok choy)
- Blackstrap molasses
- Fish with soft, edible bones, such as salmon and sardines. (Do not offer these to young children because of the choking hazard.) Blenderizing these and mixing them into casseroles and soups may help (if necessary) mask their use, as well as lower the risk for choking.

Strategies for Consuming Dairy Products:

- Drink milk in small amounts, such as 2-4 ounce servings

- Consume dairy products as part of a meal, never alone
- Consume fermented dairy products, such as refrigerated yogurt with live, active cultures, cottage cheese, and hard, aged cheese (preferably aged over five years, such as cheddar or swiss). Also try frozen yogurt with live, active cultures

Keep in mind, supplementation of calcium, vitamin D, and magnesium may be necessary depending on your child's ability to tolerate and accept dairy products and other calcium sources and should be discussed with your physician or a registered dietitian. Once lactose intolerance is resolved, it should be safe for your child to resume consuming lactose without any limitations. Some children, however, have a permanent lactose intolerance that requires lifelong lactose modification.

Sucrose and Maltose Intolerance

Physicians do not usually look for sucrase and maltase deficiencies as often as they look for lactase deficiency. Children with celiac disease, however, can have one or both of these deficiencies.

As with lactose intolerance, some physicians will simultaneously biopsy for sucrase and maltase deficiency when they are doing the biopsy to diagnose celiac disease. This part of the biopsy is generally sent out to a special laboratory for evaluation. Hydrogen breath testing is an alternative method to determine these deficiencies.

If the doctor doesn't perform one of these tests, he or she must rely on the characteristic symptoms to determine whether a deficiency is likely. For example, you or your child might notice that he has diarrhea, cramps, and/or nausea after consuming gluten-free, sweet food or any gluten-free, carbohydrate-rich foods. If other non- or low-carbohydrate, gluten-free foods, such as meat and nuts, do *not* cause similar symptoms, your child may indeed have an intolerance to these particular disaccharides.

How should this be treated? Since sweet foods, such as candy bars, sodas, and juice drinks do not contribute to good nutrition, you can eliminate or cut down on their consumption. Your child may also need to reduce or eliminate some nutritious carbohydrate foods, such as bread and cereal products. Actually, smaller, frequent meals are often better tolerated at first by anyone who has a new diagnosis of celiac disease. As the intestinal mucosa heals, normal disaccharidase levels return and your child should have no further need for dietary modification.

Your Growing Vegetarian

Many preteens and teens experiment with some type of vegetarianism as they explore and test the limits of their independence and self-expression. In addition, many families convert to vegetarianism in pursuit of a healthier lifestyle or in hopes of preventing various chronic diseases.

With appropriate guidance, knowledge, and effort it is possible to meet the specific nutritional requirements of your growing vegetarian with celiac disease. In fact, a vegetarian diet could actually be more nutritious and healthful than the typical adolescent diet, which is often high in calories, protein, and fat, and low in complex carbohydrates, including fiber, and in minerals.*,** To ensure that your child's diet is healthful, however, you, the parent, will need to be supportive, and your adolescent should be genuinely motivated and prefer eating vegetarian foods. In addition, both you and your child need to be knowledgeable about basic nutrition principles.

Vegetarian diets are based on plant foods and omit animal products to varying degrees. They run the gamut from *lacto-ovovegetarianism,* which includes foods from the dairy group and eggs, to strict vegetarianism (a *vegan* diet), which eliminates all animal products.

Whenever an entire food group is eliminated from the diet, there is the potential for nutrient deficiencies. Because of this risk, as well as the possibility that too few calories will be consumed, I personally do not recommend strict vegetarianism, especially in children with celiac disease. However, if your child wants to try a vegan diet, it is vital for him to get nutrition counseling from a registered dietitian experienced in celiac disease and vegetarianism.

Nutritional Concerns

Getting Enough Calories. It is absolutely essential that your child consume enough calories for energy and enough nutrients to promote normal development and growth—as well as to catch up growth, if necessary. For several reasons, however, it can be more difficult for vegetarians to consume the calories and nutrients they need:

- Vegetarianism usually results in higher fiber consumption, which can satisfy hunger in children too quickly.
- If too much fiber is consumed, it can interfere with the absorption of minerals, such as calcium, iron, and zinc, as well as magnesium and copper.
- This, along with the reduction or total elimination of animal products, can result in inadequate calories. If this happens, your child's growth will be affected as protein is then used for energy rather than for growth and tissue repair.

---

* Mariani, P., M. Viti, M. Montuori, A. La Vecchia, E. Cipolletta, and L. Calvani. "The Gluten-Free Diet: A Nutritional Risk Factor for Adolescents with Celiac Disease?" *Journal of Pediatric Gastroenterology and Nutrition* 1998; 27:519-523.

** Polito, C., A. Olivieri, L. Marchese, G. Desired, F. Pullano, and F. Rea. "Weight Overgrowth of Coeliac Children on Gluten-Free Diet." *Nutrition Research* 1992; 12:353-358.

To prevent these problems from occurring, it is important to provide a balance (depending on your child's age) of cooked and raw fruits and vegetables. Balancing whole grains with refined enriched bread and cereal products is also important. Legumes, nuts, and seeds also need to be incorporated into this balancing act. To estimate the range of fiber your child needs, here is a simple calculation you can use: From age 2 through 18, add your child's age to a range of 5 grams/day of fiber to 10 grams/day*. For example, a 5-year-old needs 10 to 15 grams of fiber each day.

Getting Enough Amino Acids. Another important concern for vegetarians is getting enough amino acids. We all need amino acids, whether we are vegetarian or not. They are the building blocks of protein. While the body makes *nonessential* amino acids, it must obtain *essential* amino acids from food sources in order to make the protein used for growth and tissue production.

All the essential amino acids are supplied by meat, poultry, and seafood (which are eliminated in vegetarian diets); the dairy group; eggs; and soybean protein (which may also need to be modified or totally eliminated due to a soy sensitivity/allergy). Foods containing protein of lower quality, such as legumes, nuts, seeds, and bread and cereal products supply some, but not all, of the essential amino acids. In the past, it was believed that vegetarians should combine different types of these foods in the same meal so as to consume all of the essential amino acids at once. Now, however, we know that these kinds of foods (with lower quality protein) need only be eaten over the course of the day. As long as your child eats adequate, varied, age-appropriate, nutritious meals and snacks every day, his requirements for essential amino acids, as well as protein quantity, can be satisfied.

Avoiding Nutrient Deficiencies. Without careful food selection and/ or the use of vitamin and mineral supplementation, vegetarians can develop nutrient deficiencies. These can include deficiencies of vitamins A, D, calcium, iron, zinc, vitamin B12 (cobalamin), and vitamin B2 (riboflavin).

It may be challenging to get adequate iron when sources of heme iron (meat, poultry, and seafood) are eliminated. However, vegetarians tend to consume relatively more vitamin C, which improves their iron absorption. Menstruation increases the need for iron consumption, making it especially important for teenaged girls to eat sufficient amounts of legumes, nuts, seeds, whole grains, and enriched bread and cereal products.

Animal products are naturally the only source of vitamin B12. This means a lacto-ovovegetarian or lactovegetarian (one who consumes dairy products, not eggs) should be able to satisfy their need for this vitamin. However, for a vegan, consuming enough vitamin B12 is a concern. Some foods that a vegan might typically eat, such as vitamin B12-fortified soy beverages, are a reliable source. If

---

* "Kids: They're Not Little Adults." National Dairy Council. 1996.

a vegan cannot satisfy his requirements for this important vitamin from fortified foods, he will eventually require vitamin B12 supplementation. Incidentally,
vegans may require supplementation of vitamin D (depending on the quality
and quantity of sunlight exposure), and the need for supplementation of calcium, iron, and zinc should also be evaluated.

Easy and Tasty Vegetarian Meals

There are some popular, child-pleasing entrees that naturally omit meat,
poultry, and seafood. These include beans and rice, corn tortilla with refried beans
as in a tostada or meatless taco, meatless chili with a cornbread muffin, and pasta
faggioli (pasta and beans). Not only do these combinations please the taste buds
while supplying all the essential amino acids, they are *easy* to prepare. Using
dried canned beans is just as good as soaking and cooking dried beans yourself.
Other favorites that can be easily prepared vegetarian style include stir-fries, pasta
dishes, casseroles, soups, stews, burritos, polenta dishes, and muffins and quick
breads baked with nuts or seeds.

Acquiring vegetarian recipes and cookbooks will help you satisfy the nutritional needs of your growing vegetarian. Bette Hagman's *The Gluten-free Gourmet
Cooks Fast and Healthy* offers some recipes. The American Institute of Cancer
Research provides one free copy of their booklet "Moving Towards a Plant-based
Diet: Menus and Recipes for Cancer Prevention." See the Resource Guide in the
back of the book for ordering information. For free information on how to use
beans and for recipes, write to the Michigan Bean Commission at the address in
the Resource Guide. Recipes and information on how to use tofu and other soybean products may be obtained online at www.soyfoods.com or www.talksoy.com
or by calling 1-800-TALK SOY.

Keep in mind that all the vegetarian recipes you obtain will not be gluten-
free. Many of those that are not, however, can easily be modified to be so.

Making Snacks Count

Beware! Danna's chapter on junk food is enough to make any registered
dietitian's stomach turn, as well as your child's if he eats too much junk. If you are
more nutrition conscious, read on.

It is important that children of all ages snack. In fact, we metabolize food
better when we eat smaller quantities more frequently. Unfortunately, snacking is
too often treated as a time to fill children with empty calorie foods, void of anything healthful to the human body. Junk food in moderation is acceptable, but
when excessive can wreak havoc.

Snacks should not be provided haphazardly, but rather planned and used to
meet your child's nutritional needs. This is especially important in adolescence,

when many teens eat only an evening meal and snack frequently. Snacks, like meals, should be eaten in an established place, such as the kitchen, patio, or outside play area. Because of their small stomachs and high activity level, toddlers need to eat approximately every two to three hours. Consequently, if there is a prolonged period of time between meals, offer the toddler two snacks between each meal, spaced apart. Early school-age children usually need one or two snacks a day, while the need to snack varies in older children and adolescents.

Snacks should be eaten at a given time so as not to interfere with the mealtime appetite. Usually snacks are less likely to spoil your child's appetite if eaten at least one and a half to two hours before a meal. If your child is voracious and eats a large snack, thereby suppressing his appetite for the next meal, have him snack earlier. Remind him that you do not want the snack to interfere with the next meal and establish a time limit for finishing the snack. If you have a toddler or preschooler, do not allow him to gulp sippy cups of juice all day. This acts as a continuous snack, and children who do this routinely tend not to be "good eaters."

Children of any age should not be allowed to "graze" all day or receive food handouts whenever they demand. Also discourage snacking while playing. Otherwise, you may find your child eating out of boredom and getting less than ideal nutrient consumption. Finally, using food handouts to divert, calm, or amuse your child teaches him to identify food as a panacea, which can lead to overeating and food addiction.

Parents should encourage and model nutritious snacking. Remember, those who purchase the food are the gatekeepers. If you bring nutritious snacks into the house, they will likely be eaten. Your child is more apt to accept snacks that you and he have jointly decided to purchase (ideally through use of the Food Guide Pyramid).

Examples of nutritious snacks include:
- pizza bagels or pizza rice cakes
- cheese (string cheese is a favorite) and crackers
- crackers and nut or seed butters
- refrigerated or frozen yogurt
- ice cream
- pudding, rice or bread pudding
- frozen juice bars
- fresh fruit (for example, what kid can resist grapes? Be sure to chop or slice them lengthwise for infants and toddlers)
- trail mix/gorp
- dried fruit such as apricots, pears, and raisins
- popcorn
- muffins
- cereal and milk or milk alternative

School-age children or adolescents experiencing peer pressure are more likely to eat gluten-free snacks that are similar to the gluten-containing ones their peers eat. These may include bagels, soft pretzels, hard pretzels, baked tortilla chips, and granola bars.

If your child eats too many junk food snacks, the best course is probably to let him know that you disapprove and remind him of the snacks the two of you had agreed upon and purchased. Getting into a fight over this is probably not worthwhile. You could end up with a strained relationship, and your child might feel less secure in openly asking for help about other issues.*

Managing Food Jags

A food jag refers to a phase when a child requests or demands a particular food or foods (generally for no specific reason) over others, then later adamantly refuses to eat this food and prefers a different food.** It is also considered a food jag if a child wants to eat the same food or only a few foods, such as hot dogs, for all three meals over a period of time.*** Food jags, as abnormal as they seem to parents, tend to occur at some point in all children. They often begin at approximately age one and can occur sporadically through the toddler years. They can, however, occur at any age.

Interestingly, I have often observed food jags becoming less frequent after a child has been diagnosed with celiac disease and has embarked on the gluten-free lifestyle. Prior to diagnosis, many a child is enticed by his unknowing parents to eat gluten-infested foods. Instinctively, the child rejects food because of the effects its gluten content has on his body. Then, as gluten begins to clear out of the gastrointestinal tract, more desirable eating patterns become habit.

What should you do when your child has food jags? There are various approaches. First and foremost, do not allow yourself to become emotional. This may be especially difficult if your child is not healthy and you realize that food is the source of his medical condition. It may actually please your child if he sees that he can have that much control over you, his parent.

If food jags seem to be a way of life, do not discuss feeding techniques or food while eating. Steer meal conversations onto pleasant subjects other than food.

Whatever you do, do not leave bowls and plates of any kind of food around the house to get your child to eat. This does not work! This form of "grazing" hinders the normal physiological desire for food because a true sense of hunger is not experienced or satisfied by eating.

---

* Satter, E. *How to Get Your Kid to Eat... But Not Too Much.* Palo Alto, CA: Bull Publishing, 1987.

** Satter, E. *How to Get Your Kid to Eat... But Not Too Much.* Palo Alto, CA: Bull Publishing, 1987.

*** Broihier, C. "Do You Have a Picky Eater at Home?" *Nutrition Education for the Public.* A Practice Group of The American Dietetic Association. 1993.

You may want to accommodate your child's request for a particular food or foods, but also serve him a small amount, such as one tablespoon each, of other foods. Letting your child choose a meal or snack at which he can eat his favorite food is another technique.

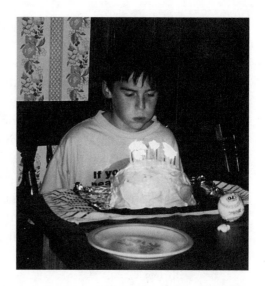

Involve your child in the family meal planning and preparation when possible. Then have him eat what everyone else does on the grounds that it is gluten free. If your child refuses to eat what is served, excuse him from the table and give him water to drink until the designated snack time. If he asks for a cookie or cracker, be firm with your limits and expectations and remind him that he must wait until snack time. Being consistent with this approach will eventually teach him that mealtime is for eating and for eating meals, not "munchies." When snack time does come, it is all the more important to provide nutritious snacks. Another technique is to calmly cover and refrigerate your child's meal if he initially refuses to eat it. Later, when he is hungry, reheat and serve it to him. (This method is very effective in our home.) It also teaches a lesson in preventing waste.

If a food jag persists for more than one to two weeks, it is a good idea to consult your physician or a registered dietitian about providing multivitamin and mineral supplementation. This can compensate for the potential lack of nutrient consumption, as well as malabsorption due to celiac disease.

Boosting Calories and Nutrients in Your Child's Diet

Is your child malnourished or nearing this mark, food "jagging," or just plain finicky? If so, you may feel challenged to get him to eat more calories and/or nutrients. The following ideas should help you achieve your goal of improving his nutritional status. While using many of these ideas, your child will not even be aware that you are working toward such a goal.

For Added Calories
- Add cooking oil, butter, or margarine (1 teaspoon provides 45 calories) to baby food, cooked cereal, cooked vegetables, rice, potatoes, soups, casseroles, and pasta dishes.

- Spread cooking oil, then mayonnaise on bread when making a sandwich.
- Add mayonnaise (1 tablespoon provides 135 calories) to salad dressing or cook into scrambled eggs. Spread it thick onto sandwiches.
- Polycose (a liquid and powder form of corn-based carbohydrate made by Ross Medical Nutritional Line) may be added to any liquid, such as juice or milkshakes, or to soft, blended type foods, such as pudding, yogurt, cooked cereal, or mashed potatoes.
- Add honey to cream cheese or ricotta cheese and use as a dip or spread. *Note: Never give honey in any form—raw, cooked, or baked—during the first year of life!* It can have clostridium botulinum spores, which can cause botulism, a serious and potentially life-threatening illness.
- Spread jam/jelly on thick.

For Added Calories and Nutrients

- Offer dried fruit alone or sprinkle over salads, cooked vegetables, or cereal; mix into a dip, ice cream, or yogurt; or use in place of, or with, jam/jelly on peanut butter sandwiches.
- Serve canned fruit packed in heavy syrup.
- Mix blackstrap molasses into baked beans, yogurt smoothies, cooked cereal, or nut or seed butters and spread on toast/bread, pancakes, waffles, French toast, or crepes.
- Add enriched rice baby cereal to blenderized food, blended yogurt and fruit smoothies, milkshakes, meatballs, or meatloaf and use as breading for meat, poultry, and fish.
- Sprinkle gluten-free granola or crumble gluten-free granola bars over fruit purees, such as applesauce. Eat "as is" or heat.

For Added Calories and Nutrients Including Protein

- Consider increasing the calorie and nutrient content of infant formula from the standard 20 calorie/ounce formulation to a more calorie- and nutrient-concentrated form. Be sure your pediatrician is aware of this modification. He or a public health registered dietitian or hospital pediatric registered dietitian can provide directions on how to make this change.
- Make double milk by mixing 1 cup of liquid milk, such as whole milk, with 1/3 cup of instant nonfat dry milk. The result is a more nutritious, rich-tasting cup of milk that can be used to drink, to make pudding, and to replace water in soups, cooked cereal, and hot

chocolate. If your child has lactose intolerance but can tolerate a small amount of lactose, an alternative beverage, such as soy or almond beverage, can be used in place of the liquid milk.

- Add instant nonfat dry milk or soymilk powder to cooked cereal, yogurt, soup, stew, mashed potatoes, cookie and muffin recipes, meatballs, meatloaf, and ground meat/poultry for burgers.
- Sprinkle shredded cheese or parmesan cheese on bread, then toast in toaster oven.
- Sprinkle cheese on baked white potatoes, sweet potatoes or yams, soups, stews, meats, salads, cooked vegetables, as well as salads.
- Add eggs to casseroles such as macaroni and cheese (before they are cooked/baked), and use extra eggs in omelets.
- Mix yogurt into fruit salad and dry cereal with or without milk, and use as a topping on pie, pancakes, waffles, or French toast.
- Offer health/energy bars. They make a great substitute for a candy bar.
- Besides peanut butter, use nut and seed butters for sandwiches and crackers. Also spread on fresh fruit, such as apples and strawberries, mix into dry cereal with milk or cooked cereal, and incorporate into the recipes of rice cereal treats.
- Serve Boost Pudding (made by Mead Johnson) and Ensure Pudding (made by Ross Medical Nutritional Line).

For More Guidance

If you have any questions or concerns about your child's nutrition that this chapter doesn't answer, it would be wise to consult a registered dietitian (R.D.) who is experienced with children (pediatrics) and celiac disease. A registered dietitian is an expert in food and nutrition with a minimum of at least a bachelor's degree in the area of these disciplines. To use the title "registered dietitian," an individual must complete a preprofessional internship or field experience and pass a national exam. To maintain these credentials, continuing education credits must be obtained.

In contrast, the title "nutritionist" can be used by anyone who chooses to define himself as such. A nutritionist may or may not be adequately educated in the field of food and nutrition. Some registered dietitians, however, have a job title of nutritionist. What is important to note is whether the individual with the title nutritionist has the R.D. credential.

To find a registered dietitian in your area, contact any of the national or local support groups for celiac disease. Some of these have registered dietitians associated with them. Also, the American Dietetic Association (A.D.A.) offers a referral service that can help you locate a registered dietitian in a given area with particular specialties. The A.D.A. may be contacted by calling 1-800-366-1655 or entering their website at *www.eatright.org*.

24

Your Family's Emotional Well-Being

Margaret V. Austin, Ph.D.

Throughout this book, parents are urged to "Deal with it; don't dwell on it." This is excellent advice if you can take it. However, as Chapter Three touched on, there are a number of emotions that can overwhelm parents and their children with celiac disease after the initial diagnosis, and coping with them is not always straightforward. In addition, some of these emotions may resurface months or years after you thought you had vanquished them. Some families simply take more time to cope with these emotions, while others need more guidance and information. For these people, the information in this chapter is meant to elaborate and enhance the information related to the emotional impact of the diagnosis found earlier in the book.

The Three Stages of Adjustment

Children and their families usually go through three broad stages in adjusting to and managing the diagnosis of celiac disease:

1. Initial shock and adjustment,
2. Ongoing management and maintenance, and
3. Periodic relapse and the recurring wish that things were different.

This chapter will attempt to outline some specific pointers for parents in helping both themselves and their children cope during each of these stages. As explained below, what impact each of these phases has on your child will depend on her age or developmental stage at diagnosis. What you can do to help your child and yourself cope will also depend somewhat on your child's age. The information about helping children cope is therefore designed to address differences in children of different ages diagnosed with celiac disease.

The Initial Shock and Adjustment Phase

Shortly after the diagnosis, your family must deal with the shock of the news, try to make lifestyle changes, and develop a new routine that manages the dietary changes. How long you stay in this phase can vary significantly according to individual temperaments, the dynamics of your family, and the age of your child at diagnosis.

During this stage, a range of uncomfortable emotions may arise because you feel a sensation of loss. For example, perhaps you feel as if you have lost the image you had for your child's future. Or perhaps you feel that you have lost the ability to protect your child from harm. The specific meaning of the diagnosis to individual families varies widely. Many families, though, could benefit from giving some thought as to what exactly the diagnosis means to them.

According to Elisabeth Kübler-Ross, who has written extensively on how people adjust to death and other losses, a loss of any kind typically requires that people go through a period of mourning and adjustment in order to integrate the new information and circumstance into their existing mental framework. This can be painful, but ultimately rewarding. Kübler-Ross lists the emotions that will most likely arise during a period of grief as:

- Denial,
- Anger,
- Bargaining,
- Despair, and
- Acceptance.

The adjustment phase can last anywhere from the first six months to the first several years following diagnosis of celiac disease (or another significant health concern). When families spend more time in this phase, it may be because they have trouble adapting to either the gluten-free lifestyle or the associated emotions. Some people simply take longer to fully accept such difficult news. They may need to put more time and effort into adjusting to negative news of any sort than some other people do. Once they have adjusted, however, these people/families may actually maintain a more consistently successful lifestyle management program. So, just because it takes your family awhile to adapt doesn't mean you won't be very successful at helping your child live a happy, healthy life.

Emotions during the Adjustment Phase

Kübler-Ross has found that most people do not move smoothly and sequentially through the stages of grief. It is more likely that people will move back and forth between the various emotions and may spend extended time in one stage or another. Grieving is a complex process, complicated further by the fact that loss of any kind tends to rekindle emotions related to the person's experience of earlier losses. This means the grieving process is highly individualized, and the time it takes varies greatly from person to person.

Parents' Emotions
Conflicting Emotions and Panic

Following the initial diagnosis of celiac disease, each parent is likely to experience a range of emotions, including both relief at finally having an answer to the ongoing concerns about their child's health and panic related to what will happen now. In addition to the conflicting emotions, implications of the diagnosis and concerns about lifestyle management begin to rapidly arise. In fact, the whole situation can feel extremely overwhelming.

Each of the numerous issues that arise must be sorted through and dealt with before moving on. Luckily, not everything has to be done the same day. It is important to realize that the panic you feel at first is a normal part of the adaptation process, and *it will pass.*

Denial

Because having a child diagnosed with a serious illness is extremely painful, many parents may experience a sense of denial in response to their child's diagnosis. This may take the form of seeking a second opinion (which is often a wise response to any serious diagnosis, anyway); refusing to change the family's eating habits and observing their child's response to specific meals; or challenging the diagnosis by changing their child's diet, reintroducing forbidden foods, and observing the child's reactions. However it is expressed, denial is a normal response to loss, and it is, by definition, a phase because the truth of the matter can only be avoided for so long. However, once the facts are in, it is important for parents to intentionally move themselves quickly through this stage because their actions (what they feed their child) can have a dramatic impact on their child's health.

It is also quite common for denial to become an issue again a few months after the child has been on a gluten-free diet and is beginning to look and feel much better. Many parents begin to suspect that perhaps there was never really anything wrong in the first place! To complicate matters further, many parents who challenge their child's diet after the first biopsy and before the second notice that their child doesn't show any response to gluten. This may also occur when a child inadvertently eats gluten. Unfortunately, this is typical for many children with celiac disease and does not indicate that the child is problem free. It is more likely that the child's body is reacting to the gluten in a manner that is difficult to see. In many cases, there must be a build-up of gluten to trigger observable symptoms. Remember that this condition does not tend to be overdiagnosed and people with celiac disease do not grow out of it, so it is extremely unlikely that the diagnosis will change.

Denial is a powerful emotion that tends to arise repeatedly, and the lack of immediate gluten-related response may even encourage it. You will need to address denial each time it arises, because your child's health will suffer if you give in to denial.

Anger

According to Kübler-Ross, anger is the next difficult emotion that is likely to be experienced in response to a loss. The anger experienced may be entirely irrational in that the target of the anger may not be clearly identified, or if it is identified, it may not make logical sense to be angry at the target. For example, some people may be angry at God for allowing their child to become ill. Others are even angry at the ancestor that passed the "defective gene" to their child. This type of anger is likely to be very powerful, may not be clearly understood, and may be free floating. The anger is likely to be so strong because it is the current emotional focal point of all emotions related to this issue. In other words, the various emotions experienced, at least for a time, become lumped together under the guise of anger. This feature also explains why anger is often not clearly understood. How does anyone rationally understand that the experience of anger becomes the center point for all emotions related to the child's recent diagnosis? This process is difficult to fathom, especially when one is in the midst of the anger.

If you are in the grip of free-floating anger, anger is the underlying emotion being experienced almost all of the time regardless of the context or the company. You are likely to have a very short temper, becoming angry easily and in response to events that normally would not trigger anger. Therefore, anger may be the emotional state in the grieving process that other people find the most difficult to handle. People who are this angry are likely to behave in a manner that pushes others away, even those who are trying to be helpful. If you remain in this stage for an extended period, you may therefore have problems in numerous relationships during this time.

Bargaining

The term bargaining refers to the somewhat desperate tendency to dream up wild hopes that somehow a certain action could change the reality of the diagnosis. After going through the denial and the anger phases, many people still remain unconvinced of the true situation. They may dwell on unrealistic courses of action (such as if I could only wake from this nightmare). Or they may try almost magical thinking (such as, if I only avoid white flour, my child will have no further problems with gluten). They may invest a situation with power it doesn't have (such as, if I see another doctor, she or he will discover my child's true diagnosis and it will be easy to remedy). Some people bargain with God to intervene (such as, I will never drink again, if you will only cure my child).

These types of bargaining represent the last desperate efforts to avoid facing the diagnosis. People in this stage of the grieving process may move quickly through it, easily recognizing the futility of such hopes. Others may need to actually take some of the actions in order to test whether or not the result is as they hope. Either way, this phase is a natural part of the grieving process and should not be considered a setback for either those experiencing it or those trying to support them through the difficult times.

Despair

Most parents do experience sadness and grief when their child is diagnosed with celiac disease. Although grief is a very normal response to any perceived loss, that fact alone does not make it any easier to deal with. You may feel sad because you worry that your child may experience difficulties in life because of this diagnosis, that her life won't be absolutely perfect, or that she may be teased or experience health problems. In addition, there are many changes ahead: in your view of your child, in your child's view of herself, and in the lifestyle that you all probably took for granted.

The diagnosis of a child with a serious health condition is no doubt one of life's biggest challenges. It is entirely normal to experience sadness and grief at this prospect. However, unlike with the death of a child, despair may be too strong a response to this news. Often, by this time in the grieving process, parents have begun a gluten-free diet and are thankful that their child's health is improving. For some people, this may be enough to send them down the adaptation trail. Others may be profoundly sad and face more of a challenge in moving on.

Regardless of its intensity, sadness is likely to be a recurring emotion for most people throughout the adaptation process.

Acceptance

This phase in the grieving process refers to the time in which your mental framework begins to shift and you are able to begin accepting the new situation. You will know you have reached this stage if brief thoughts about celiac disease no longer immediately bring you to denial, anger, or despair.

By now you will have witnessed your child's improvement in response to the gluten-free diet and will be starting to glimpse the fact that life will go on in the face of this diagnosis. Your child *will* laugh, play, go to school and other events, play sports, and even eat despite her inability to tolerate gluten. This realization is the proverbial light at the end of the tunnel and the light will grow as you begin to spend more time in this stage of grieving and less time in the others. There is more to life than eating, and once you can begin to recognize this, you are well on your way to acceptance.

The goal of the grieving process is to reach this stage and become firmly entrenched here. Of course, there will be times when managing the challenge of raising a celiac child will be more difficult than others. Negative emotions will most likely resurface from time to time. However, once you are able to get off the emotional roller coaster and consistently manage the required lifestyle changes in a matter-of-fact style, you are ready to move into the Management and Maintenance phase (see below).

What to Do for Yourself

The first thing parents can do for themselves is to recognize that they *are* grieving and allow themselves a grieving period. Again, the specific length of time required here will vary significantly from person to person. Whatever the time frame, it is important to be patient with yourself just as you would do for your child or someone else you care about. Grieving does take time and attention. Ignoring your feelings will not help the situation and in fact could hurt it. Remember that difficult emotions tend to become more manageable when dealt with directly than they are when ignored. However, it is also important not to dwell on your grief.

Finding a comfortable balance between ignoring your emotions and dwelling on them is a difficult challenge. Two possible signs that you may be dwelling on your grief are that you are either unable to complete daily tasks or are having ongoing or repeated destructive thoughts. Remember that needing emotional support from others is not a weakness; it is a step toward regaining strength. Don't be afraid of asking for help from significant others or from a professional if you feel the need.

Coping with Panic: The panic phase usually doesn't last very long. Few people can maintain emotions of such intensity for extended periods. However, a sense of being overwhelmed can continue for quite some time. Some helpful techniques for managing feelings of being overwhelmed are:

1. Seek emotional support (it always helps to have someone to talk to).
2. Consciously choose to let go of tasks that you would normally do, but that aren't really necessary.
3. Make lists to increase your efficiency.
4. Try to break necessary tasks down into more manageable pieces (this usually helps in clarifying what actually has to be done and demonstrating that you are making progress).
5. Seek help with specific tasks (let your mother visit, ask your spouse to do something in particular, or hire someone to do specific tasks).
6. Take steps to reduce anxiety (exercise, meditate, take hot baths, etc.).

Coping with Denial: The sense of denial that many people go through also does not tend to last for a long period. The reality of a sick child and the possibility of making her worse by feeding her the wrong things usually encourages people to start making the necessary changes pretty quickly. If you are not sure whether you are in a state of denial:

1. Talk to other people (this may be difficult because some other involved people may be in denial themselves).
2. Search yourself as to what you know versus how you feel about it.
3. Most importantly, observe your child to see whether she improves on a gluten-free diet or, if she is not yet on the diet, for her response to gluten containing food.
4. Whether or not you are in denial, you, like many parents, may need more information in order to comfortably proceed. Some suggestions in proceeding with information gathering are:
   - Get a second opinion.
   - Talk to other parents whose children have also been diagnosed.
   - Read all the information you can get your hands on in order to learn about the disease and its symptoms.
   - Some doctors support parents in "challenging" the diet in order to demonstrate the accuracy of the diagnosis (be cautious with this one).
   - Make a list of all the reasons why the diagnosis seems to fit for your child and another list of the reasons it does not. Seeing the comparison written on paper may make the conclusion clear.

Coping with Anger: Anger is an emotion that is difficult for most people to deal with. People tend to avoid conflict more than any other type of situation.

This is because anger makes us uncomfortable—at least partly because we don't know how to deal with it. Nevertheless, it's important to recognize that you are angry (if you are) and acknowledge it as a normal part of the grieving process. The following suggestions may be helpful in dealing with anger.

1. Develop appropriate outlets for anger. Trying to ignore or suppress anger is never a good idea since this may build pressure and lead to outbursts. Many people prefer to deal with anger intellectually and may benefit from some type of artistic outlet such as writing in a journal or drawing a picture that represents an aspect of the problem. Others feel better if they have someone to talk to about the concerns on their mind or use some kind of physical release such as sports or exercise. Base your approach on your own style.

2. Try simply throwing yourself actively into the problem at hand, focusing on the specific tasks that must be accomplished. Problem-solving activity itself can help reduce stress and relieve anger.

3. Believe it or not, laughter can help release feelings of anger and frustration. Besides, if you can laugh at a situation, you can start to take some control at managing it. Work to maintain appreciation for the quirks of life.

4. Try to focus your anger appropriately. Random angry outbursts can distance others and add problems to the existing ones.

5. Whatever your coping style, be sure to put some effort into taking care of yourself. You will need to be stable yourself in order to be the guiding force for the changes in your child's life. Both you and your child will benefit from the time you spend maintaining and supporting yourself during this stressful time.

Coping with Despair: Despair is a particularly challenging emotion, if it is an issue at all. This may also be the emotional state that grieving people are most likely to become stuck in. Nevertheless, even in the midst of this emotional state, there are things you can do for yourself.

1. Be sure to take care of yourself: Eat nutritional meals and get plenty of rest. Avoid alcohol or drugs, as they may increase feelings of grief.

2. Reach out to others. People with solid social relationships tend to be happier overall and to be more effective at managing difficult times.

3. Put some time into writing down a "gratitude inventory"—a list of all the things that make your life worthwhile. Include people, places, aspects of yourself, anything you can think of. Then, review this list at least daily to remind yourself of all that is good in your life.

4. Laugh at every opportunity you have. Remember that research actually indicates that laughter is good for the body as well as the

soul. It helps reduce tension, diminish fear, promote healing, and build rapport with others.

5. Exercise! Though this may be the furthest thing from your mind right now, even walking for half an hour a day can increase the body's natural endorphins, which can significantly help in managing stress and sadness.

6. Remember to relax. These negative thoughts and emotions should gradually fade as you *and* your child become more comfortable with the diet and begin to realize that a "normal life" is made up of much more than food.

7. Be aware of your sadness. If you believe that your feelings are becoming too much to bear or you begin to have frequent and repeated destructive thoughts, seek professional help. Every community has professionals in the helping field who can work with you to overcome any dark emotional cloud.

Acceptance: Moving into the acceptance phase of grieving is usually a blessed relief to most parents. There are a few things you need to do to help yourself during this phase. You should congratulate yourself for reaching this point and bask in the glow of relief. It is important to try and fully experience the moment because you want the sense of optimism often felt here to grow. Optimism can encourage resiliency, enthusiasm, and a sense of joy. There will still be difficult times ahead, but your tasks now are to appreciate yourself and your child, as well as all the good things in your life. There is nothing quite like a taste of difficult times to enhance one's appreciation for the good times.

Helping Your Child Adapt

Now it is time to discuss how children react to, and cope with, the diagnosis of celiac disease. Some parents may wonder why it has taken so long to get to the children. After all, they are the group most affected, right?

Actually, because parents are responsible for their child and have a greater level of understanding, they may be more affected than the children themselves, at least initially. Also, remember that it is the parents who guide their children through adaptation to the diagnosis and set the stage for successful lifestyle management. The more successful the parent's adaptation to the diagnosis, the more successful the child's will be. Therefore, the impact of the diagnosis on both the parent and the child is important to understand.

As mentioned above, the impact of each adjustment phase may differ significantly according to the age of your child. Since the developmental tasks of children in different age groups vary, this section will be broken down into five age groups: the very young child, the toddler, the preschool age child, the latency age child, and the teenager.

The Very Young Child

This section describes children from infancy through preschool age or about five years old. Ideally, most children with celiac disease would be diagnosed during this age range. An early diagnosis definitely makes the initial adaptation phase easier for the child.

The Infant

An infant (birth to one year), although actively learning and growing, will not be aware of any dietary changes or restrictions. Clearly, if they have been ill in relation to gluten consumption, they will begin to feel healthier following gluten restriction.

The Toddler

Toddlers (age one to two and a half years) are more aware of their environment and may notice some changes to their diet, particularly restrictions. They will also be tuned in to their parents and will react to any negativity in relation to the new diet. To help your child more successfully adapt:

1. Set a good example; act in a positive and upbeat manner. Keep your concerns and negative emotions to yourself for expression in other situations.

2. Provide plenty of opportunity for individual choice and expression in other realms. Toddlers are typically struggling for independence, so they are already prone to resistance. Although parents must generally be willing to allow a toddler room to express her new autonomy, you cannot allow this in the realm of food choice (unless all the choices are acceptable foods).

3. Do not limit your child's chances to express her autonomy due to your concerns about celiac disease. There is often a temptation to be overprotective. Resist this urge!

4. Read your child books about other children who have health concerns. Read the book first to ensure that it has points relevant to your child.

5. Support your child's efforts to positively deal with the restrictions or the diagnosis.

6. Encourage your child to express her feelings about celiac disease. Most children this age will have some difficulty talking about their feelings, but can draw or pretend with dolls in a manner that allows such emotional expression.

The Preschooler

Preschoolers are children from two and a half to five years of age. During this age range, children become more interested in the world beyond their homes. They are curious and eager to learn, and their language skills advance rapidly. Some tips for helping your preschooler adjust include:

1. Provide many opportunities for activities with peers, as preschoolers are highly social beings. This may create some problems for children on a special diet, since they may begin to compare their own eating habits to those of their peers. Despite this potential problem, it is through such activities that children gain mastery of their abilities, including social and emotional development, and achieve feelings of competence. Although you may feel tempted to keep your child away from activities that might make her feel unhappy about her diet, don't do it. Social activity provides an opportunity for your child to face and deal with her feelings regarding her diet.

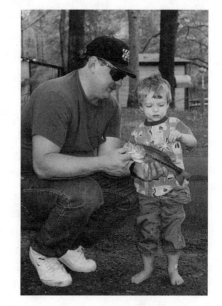

2. Remember that it is always better to face difficult issues than to suppress them. Early efforts to manage emotions help set the stage for later successful emotional and lifestyle management. Children in this age group are beginning to recognize different emotional states.

3. Help your child learn to manage her emotions. Begin by acknowledging her feelings and helping her learn to label her emotions. For example, say "I can see that you are very angry right now."

4. Encourage your child to talk about her emotions. "Can you tell me in words how angry you are?"

5. Teach your child to express her emotions appropriately. Provide some physical outlets for anger or frustration such as an obstacle course in the playroom or a bean bag that she can throw.

6. Help your child learn to maintain or regain emotional control. Stay calm, speak softly, divert attention to a soothing or fun activity, and display empathy. Be sure to express your understanding in a brief manner without adding excessive detail that may increase your child's anxiety.

7. Answer any questions your child asks about celiac disease, but do not overwhelm her with extra information. Respond only with the information necessary to satisfy her.

The Latency Age Child

Latency age refers to the period from six to twelve years of age. Children in this age group are actively learning and growing, setting the groundwork for how they will handle relationships, learning, and self-esteem in their future lives. They tend to be focused more on cooperation and belonging than do either the preschooler or the teenager. These qualities often make children in this age range much easier for parents to work with than either older or younger children.

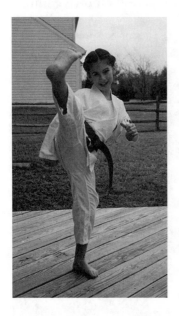

If your child is diagnosed at this age, she will definitely have a reaction to the news. She has sufficient memory of prediagnosis life to understand that she will now have to forgo many of the foods she freely ate in the past. On the other hand, because she has lived with the condition for years, she will have experienced many reactions to gluten. This means that when gluten is eliminated from her diet, she will most likely notice the improvement. This can be a very powerful motivator. Ways to help a latency age child cope include:

1. Point out how much better your child is feeling on the diet.
2. Try to demonstrate that the diagnosis is manageable and that the necessary lifestyle changes fit smoothly into the existing family format. Children from this age group will respond directly to parental efforts, both positive and negative.
3. Take care not to express a sense of being overwhelmed or depressed by the diagnosis. Some children in this age group may react by "mothering" the parent, acting as if everything is OK with them, maybe going so far to learn about the diet and implement it themselves, in an effort to encourage the parent to regroup. Others might just become depressed and overwhelmed themselves. Given this age group's tendency to try to please their parents at all cost, you need to quickly adapt to the news or at least not share any negative feelings with your child.
4. Expect your child to go through a grieving process in response to her diagnosis. Like you, she may experience conflicting feelings, including relief to know what is wrong, panic at what will happen now,

and guilt for causing her family problems. She may also experience denial: refusing to accept the diagnosis and even adamantly denying its reality despite a great deal of information to the contrary. She may wish so hard that the diagnosis isn't accurate that it may appear as if she thinks by wishing she can make it so. Next, comes the anger. Children of this age group may become tremendously angry, even if they are too young to understand the diagnosis; angry at you for taking away the foods she enjoys, or simply angry that she feels deprived. Children can easily become stuck in the anger phase and need the help and support from loving adults to facilitate moving beyond anger.

5. Encourage your child to face the difficult news, identify and discuss her feelings, and develop plans to manage the feelings and later the lifestyle changes. Your child's ability to successfully manage the grieving process largely depends on the quality of her relationship with you. Parents are the port in the storm.

6. Be sure to demonstrate respect and confidence in your child and her abilities to manage this situation.

7. Provide plenty of encouragement that actively recognizes your child's assets and strengths.

8. Make yourself available when your child needs to talk. Also be willing to facilitate talking when your child clearly needs to but can't quite find the words or the way to initiate them.

9. Finally, it is imperative to routinely demonstrate through words and actions how much you love your child. Remember that the way you relate to your children in general is the most powerful demonstration of how you feel about them. If there is a distance between you and your child or significant problems existed in your relationship prior to the diagnosis, it may help to let the diagnosis serve as a trigger to seek help to improve your relationship with your child.

The Teenager

This stage of life spans the time from about thirteen to nineteen years of age. It is a time of rapid physical development marked by a return to an increased need for autonomy and independence. Adolescents are also experimenting with all aspects of life. Emotions can be chaotic, due to hormonal changes and frequent encounters with success and failure. Teenagers seem to challenge everything; nothing is taken as a given. Rules and expectations are both valued and shunned (rules are limits, but they do provide clear guidelines). Socially, friends are becoming more important than family. Fitting in with their peer group is of paramount importance, because it is through these relationships that a sense of identity is formed. Family relationships become strained as teenagers struggle to become independent, ready or not, and parents struggle to provide the right amount of structure. In short, the teenage years are a time of confusion, experimentation, and high anxiety.

Teenagers who are diagnosed with celiac disease definitely experience the grieving response in a manner similar to their parents. They are capable of recognizing conflicting emotions, they more accurately realize the extent of the changes that will be required than do younger children, and they are more set in their ways. (Despite the age-appropriate need to challenge everything, it is only fun to challenge something if it is your own idea, not if you have to.)

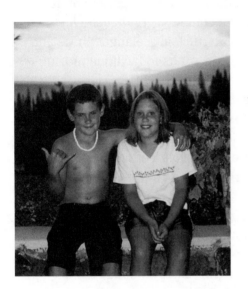

Adolescents may well become overwhelmed because of their diagnosis, but it is likely that this will change quickly into anger. Anger is often a dominant emotional state during this time period anyway. A major lifestyle change forced by a health condition is likely to generate a lot of angry energy in a rebellious teen yearning for independence. Older children may focus their anger at the same people and circumstances that adults focus on: the relative who passed on the gene, God, food manufacturers. Given the adolescent propensity for anger, this phase may last for some time.

There is also a chance that your teenager may become depressed. In fact, emotional instability is a known characteristic of the teenage years. Adolescents are frequently depressed when they get bad news in general. Being told that you have a lifelong health condition requiring you to go on a "weird," strict diet (no more cookies or cake!) may definitely strike many teenagers as a downer.

Because of all the emotions that can overwhelm a newly diagnosed teenager, it is crucial to build the best parent/teenager relationship you can. This can be hard, given the fast pace of life for teenagers and adults these days. Then, too, many teenagers want to be with their friends and resist adult intervention. With effort, though, you can help. Here are some suggestions:

1. Be willing to commit the time and attention needed to build a solid relationship.
2. Strive for clear communication, as communication problems are usually a central issue in troubled relationships. Listening to the feelings, needs, and thoughts of a child, particularly an adolescent, is

often a difficult thing for parents to do. If your teenager will even discuss her thoughts and feelings with you, it is usually a good sign.

3. Ask for clarification if you don't understand what is being said.
4. Confront the issue; don't criticize your teen. Let her know your thoughts and feelings in a way that communicates respect for her as an individual. Remember that good communication, understanding, and mutual respect are all cornerstones of healthy relationships.
5. If your teen has been recently diagnosed, keep a close eye on her emotional state. This may be a bit difficult since she may view parental concern as intrusive. However, this is very important for *all* parents of teenagers to do, whether or not they have celiac disease.
6. Watch for signs that might indicate that your child is having significant coping problems. Noticeable behavioral changes such as a sudden drop in academic performance can often indicate that a teen is in distress. Look for signs of depression such as changes in normal appetite or sleep disturbances, or personality changes such as unusual withdrawal, aggression, or moodiness.
7. Let your child know you are concerned about her.
8. Get professional help if indicated. If you believe the situation to be serious and your child refuses to seek help, arrange it for her.

The Ongoing Management and Maintenance Phase

By the time your family reaches this stage of development, you will have established a routine that is consistently followed. You will also have made some efforts to "fine tune" specific tasks within the routine and to make changes based on what works and doesn't work for your child and family. For example, your family may have started the new diet by buying all of your gluten-free bread. As you became more accustomed to making dietary modifications, you may have bought a bread maker and started baking some of your own bread. Or, your family might have started out by requiring all family members to eat gluten-free meals, but have now settled into a routine that provides both standard and gluten-free fare. At this stage, your family will have a certain amount of comfort or familiarity with the routine so that flexibility and change are possible within the overall framework of a gluten-free diet.

Most families will spend most of their time in this stage. It should last a lifetime, with occasional relapses, during which you wish that life was different.

Once a family has reached this stage, the going may be somewhat easier. The early panic and emotional turmoil have been dealt with and your family feels comfortable with its routine once again. The task ahead is simply to continue doing what works. Many families feel a sense of relief as they begin to realize that the challenge of illness and lifestyle change has been met. Success is at hand, your child with celiac disease is flourishing, and there is a sense of comfort in a familiar routine. Most people relish the realization that there is more to life than food. Families begin to relax again and the tension levels ease. Life returns to "normal"—however you defined that prior to the diagnosis. Yes, many changes have occurred, but life can now go on. Children and their families focus on all aspects of their lives, not just the dietary ones.

Periodic Relapse and Wishing That Things Were Different

This phase is not so much a stage in itself as it is a periodic part of the Ongoing Management and Maintenance stage. In other words, most children with celiac disease and their parents will remain primarily in a maintenance phase, but will periodically have behaviors or emotions from an earlier stage. Then they will quickly return to the ongoing maintenance stage. Periodic relapse should be expected and anticipated. The Ongoing Management and Maintenance stage may sound ideal because most of the major issues and the associated emotional turmoil have already been addressed. All children and families have to do is to keep on doing what they are doing. In reality, however, few people can maintain a consistently "even keel" throughout their entire life.

In fact, for many people, consistency seems to be one of the most difficult behaviors to maintain. Routines, while comfortable, can be boring, people can be tempted by other options, or children may feel angry and want to act out by eating forbidden foods in order to get back at their parents. Managing a gluten-free diet in the face of these challenges to consistency is the primary task in this stage. Luckily, these difficult times arise only periodically, and otherwise, life goes on and is full of all the things that all our lives contain: school, friends, family, work, sports, and recreation.

This stage can also be complicated by the reappearance of emotions that you believed were laid to rest. Most people experience some self-doubt, sadness, wistfulness, regret, etc. about all kinds of things at different times in their lives. For a child with celiac disease and her family, the dietary restrictions may well be a prime target for emotional upheaval.

In addition, it is human nature to readdress difficult issues that have already been faced and put to rest in the past. This tendency stems from the fact that as people grow and mature, they develop increasing knowledge, awareness, and sensitivity. These personal changes and heightened skills ideally allow individuals to address old issues in new and more sophisticated ways. Unfortunately, few of us readdress old issues intentionally. It is much more likely that we suddenly find ourselves facing an old issue that we thought we buried long ago. If you are aware of this human tendency for periodic emotional turmoil, you can anticipate its occurrence and be prepared to manage the associated challenges. It helps to realize that each time this occurs, it is an opportunity to take understanding and personal or behavioral change to greater heights. Try not to view these periodic relapses as negative, but as a part of the human need for ongoing growth.

What to Do For Yourself

Parents often feel the greatest sense of relief once they reach the Maintenance phase. Parents are likely the ones who have worried the most. Therefore, once parents catch their breath and realize that the crisis is over, it still may take some time to begin to relax. The inability to fully relax may actually be helpful because staying on the gluten-free diet does require ongoing and consistent work. Problems will always ebb and flow. Lifestyle issues aren't resolved once and for all; they require at least periodic focus and effort. This doesn't mean that parents must stay worried and tense for the rest of their lives. Rather, parents must remain ever vigilant to the possibility of problems arising; and when they do, take charge of orchestrating the resolution.

Your task is essentially to remain ready to douse fires, as necessary, and to always support your child in growing as a person. Here are some suggestions to help you fully meet this responsibility:

1. Take care of yourself! Don't think that this is selfish! Rejuvenating yourself is imperative to meeting life's demands as a parent.

2. Learn to manage living with a routine in other areas of life—daily hygiene, exercise, first housework then playtime on the weekends. The actual routine is not as important as simply learning to function consistently. Consistency is a behavior that most of us have to work toward. Parents must be able to behave consistently in order to make the necessary lifestyle changes for their family, as well as to teach their children the value of routine.

3. Provide some spice to the routine by occasionally trying something different—adding new foods to the menu or finding a new restaurant to try.

4. Maintain significant relationships with people other than your children. All of us have numerous and varied needs; no single person or relationship can possibly meet them all. An adult family member, spouse, or friend can listen to the problems you may have and support you in your efforts to solve them. Or, significant others can also happily distract you from your worries and remind you of what is wonderful in life.

The Very Young Child

During this stage, very young children will have various needs, depending on their developmental level and abilities. Tips to help your child include:

1. Target your efforts to help your child manage her diet and other lifestyle issues at her developmental level. Give some thought to allowing your child as much responsibility for her diet as possible, given her capabilities.

2. Take full control of menu planning and food preparation until your child has the ability to contribute in these areas.

3. Allow your child choices among different gluten-free foods as much as possible.

4. Maintain a calm and matter-of-fact air about the diet and the lifestyle changes. Your child will pick up on your attitudinal expressions—both positive and negative. So, keep it positive.

5. Explain as necessary to adults in your children's life. Keep these explanations positive as well, especially if your child might hear you.

6. Make special arrangements ahead of time for parties, play dates, and other activities that may involve food.

7. Be firm, but not judgmental, about your child's food consumption. Avoid making mealtime a battleground. What your child eats is up to you; whether or not she eats it and how much she eats is up to her. This will help set the stage early in your child's life that mealtime is a pleasant family time, not a time for power and control struggles.

8. Continue to work with your child on identifying and appropriately expressing her feelings. The happiest and most successful children are those who learn how to effectively deal with their emotions.

The Latency Age Child

Children in this age group, as mentioned above, are likely to be much more cooperative than either older or younger children. Keep this in mind and use it to your advantage.

1. Let your child gradually take increasing responsibility for menu planning. She knows what she likes, and will enjoy knowing that she helped with the planning.

2. If she is interested, teach your child about food preparation. She certainly needs to know how to do this, and will be more accepting of instructions at this age.

3. Remember to avoid battles over eating. Although children in this stage are generally more agreeable, they do have tempers and are only now learning to successfully manage them. As a parent, you

want to avoid making food a pawn in a power struggle between you and your child.

4. Observe your child's emotional states. She is much more likely to eat forbidden food when she is upset about something than when things are going well. Try to curb problems before they really get started.

5. Support your child in learning how to tell friends or other children who ask about her diet. Teach her that she doesn't have to talk about it just because she is asked. Tell her what she can say to avoid the topic. If she chooses to discuss it, what are the words she should use and how far should she go with the explanation? You may even want to role play various scenarios with her.

6. Support all your child's efforts to positively manage the diet or the lifestyle.

7. Remain available to help your child identify, manage, and properly express feelings, both related to her diet and any other issues or problems.

8. Maintain a close and supportive relationship with your child.

The Teenager

In many ways, teenagers are the most challenging group. Their developmental task is to begin separation from their family, yet they are still dependent on their parents for many things: both emotional and physical support, structure, appropriate limits, and ongoing help in learning to manage an increasingly complex world. Of course, there are times when they won't want their parents' support, but they need it anyway. Sticking to a routine and being consistent tend not to be easy for adolescents, yet that is exactly what they need to do to successfully manage their diets. Given all these tendencies, a parent's role is critically important and difficult to define. Here are some suggestions that may help bridge your teenager's conflicting needs for independence and parental support:

1. Avoid battles over eating. This has been important throughout your child's previous years, but given the adolescent need for independence, it is even more important (and difficult) now.

2. If eating correctly becomes an issue, remind your child of the consequences of eating forbidden food, briefly tell her that you think she should stick with the diet, and then give her room to make her own decision.

3. Demonstrate confidence in your child's ability to make the right decision.

4. If your child goes off her diet, try not to be critical or to gloat. Simply encourage her to get back into her routine as soon as possible.

5. Support all efforts to positively manage the diet or the lifestyle.

6. Continue to watch for any signs of emotional disruption and remain available for discussions and support, as needed.
7. Take active steps to maintain a close relationship with your child. Your child still needs your affection and support, even though she may not act as though she does.
8. Remember that it is up to you to ensure that lifestyle management issues are dealt with successfully. Even with teenagers, a parent's job is primarily to teach their children what they need to know to be successful in the world.

Final Thoughts

If you find yourself struggling to handle lifestyle changes or emotional issues, check out some of the numerous books available at bookstores and libraries on the grieving process and on managing specific emotional states. Support groups can also be vital to realizing that you are not alone. There are celiac support groups that may be very helpful. There may also be support groups for parents of chronically ill children, or some other offshoot that would provide useful information. There may even be support groups for children of various ages in your community. The Resource Guide at the back of the book lists some groups that are more national in scope; these groups may be able to direct you to local chapters in your area.

Another option is to join a therapy group. Therapy groups are available in most communities and can help with issues such as managing grief, anger, and lifestyle restrictions. Again, these groups are often available for people of various ages.

Above all, remember to take the time to enjoy what's good in life. As popular writer Ashleigh Brilliant has noted, "We have only two things to worry about—either that things will never get back to normal or that they already have." Either way, it can help greatly to simply adopt a cheerful attitude.

25 Legal Rights and Benefits

Throughout this book, we have emphasized that celiac disease is something that you and your child can not only learn to live with, but also to thrive with. We have focused on ways to make your child's experiences as much like any other child's as possible, and certainly have not suggested that celiac disease, by itself, is disabling in any way.

Still, there are a few instances when it *may* benefit your child to know about some of the federal laws and regulations relating to children with disabilities or serious health concerns. This is especially the case if your child happens to have a bona fide disability (such as Down syndrome, epilepsy, or attention-deficit hyperactivity disorder) in addition to celiac disease.

At School

If your child with celiac disease attends public school, there are two federal laws that may be relevant:

1. Section 504 of the Rehabilitation Act of 1973, which applies to most students with a diagnosis of celiac disease, and
2. The Individuals with Disabilities Education Act (IDEA), which applies only to students who have a disability that has an "educational impact" on their ability to learn (e.g., students with celiac disease who also have a disability such as Down syndrome, autism, epilepsy, or ADHD).

Section 504 of the Rehabilitation Act of 1973*

Section 504 of the Rehabilitation Act of 1973 states:

"No otherwise qualified individual with handicaps in the United States . . .shall solely by reason of her or his handicap, be excluded from the participation in, be denied the benefits of, or be subjected to discrimination under any program or activity receiving federal financial assistance...."

In other words, the law prohibits discrimination on the basis of disability in any program or activity receiving federal funds. Since public schools all receive federal funding, the law ensures that students with disabilities receive equal access to a public education. Private schools and childcare centers that receive any public funding must also comply with this law and its regulations.

For your child with celiac disease, the main protection this law offers is to prohibit discrimination when he is eating in a public school cafeteria.

Section 504 defines a person with a disability as any person who:

- has a physical or mental impairment that substantially limits one or more major life activities such as caring for oneself, performing manual tasks, walking, seeing, hearing, speaking, breathing, learning, and working;
- has a record of such an impairment; or
- is regarded as having such an impairment.

Related Aids and Services

Under Section 504, a school district must consider the individual needs of a child with disabilities and provide special education and related aids and services to enable that child to attend school and benefit from the program. These requirements may include the following:

- health services, including the administration of medication;
- related and supplementary aids and services for students with disabilities in order to enable them to benefit from regular or special education—for example, readers for blind students or menu information or ingredient substitution for students with food allergies.

---

* The following information has been adapted from "Students with Food Allergies: What Do the Laws Say?" published by the Food Allergy Network, Fairfax, VA.

Free and Appropriate Public Education

Section 504 requires federally funded public elementary and secondary education programs to provide a "free and appropriate public education" to students, regardless of the severity of the student's disability.

"Free education" means the parents will incur no costs. A school cannot charge parents, for example, for the cost of food or ingredient substitutions, or other services in the cafeteria to a student with dietary restrictions.

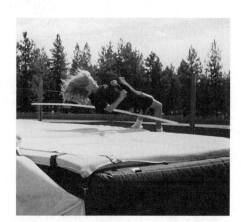

"Appropriate education" means:

- A student with a disability must be educated with nondisabled students to the extent that it is appropriate for that student.
- A student with a disability must receive access to educational opportunities or extracurricular activities equal to that provided to students without disabilities. For example, students cannot be excluded from field trips, eating in the cafeteria, or class projects because of a food allergy or celiac disease.

How Do Celiac Kids Fit into Section 504?

Section 504 requires meals to be modified for children who have a "handicapping condition" that restricts their diet, yet Section 504 does not outline how this is to be done. However, it mandates the United States Department of Agriculture (USDA) to issue instructions for State Departments of Education.

The USDA responded by including this information in the National School Lunch Act (NSLA). Under the NSLA, public schools must provide special diets for:

- Students on an "Individualized Education Program" (IEP) who have a physician's statement of need. (Children who have Down syndrome, epilepsy, or another developmental disability in addition to celiac disease would qualify under this criterion. See the next section.)
- Students with a food allergy or medical condition requiring a special diet who are not on an IEP (e.g., celiac disease, PKU, diabetes,) with a physician's statement of need.

A physician's statement of need is required to obtain a special diet at school, and must be in the student's file. (Without a doctor's note, the school can deny your request, since not all food allergies are life-threatening.) According to Joan E. Guthrie Medlen, R.D., consulting dietitian in Portland, Oregon, the physician's statement must include:

- The student's disability (celiac disease)
- The major life activity affected by the disability
- The foods to be omitted or substituted.

Medlen recommends the following steps be taken by parents who want their children to use the school's food service:

1. Obtain a statement of need that says: "(Child's name) is to be provided with a gluten-free diet per dietitian's guidelines secondary to celiac disease. Gluten will cause malabsorption and malnutrition, which will interfere with school participation." This should be written on the physician's stationery or a prescription pad, and signed by the physician.
2. Obtain a list of safe and unsafe foods from a reliable source.
3. Ask the food service staff who will review the menu to be certain it is gluten-free.
4. Ask if a registered dietitian will sign off on these menu modifications.
5. Provide a copy of the physician's statement and list of safe/unsafe foods for the child's file, the office staff, the classroom teacher(s), and the food service staff.
6. Also present this file to the school principal, and provide a copy to the school district office.

You should be aware that if the school district does not provide lunches to *any* children (there is no school lunch program in place), which happens in small, rural towns, the school cannot be required to provide a gluten-free diet to your child. Also remember that, in practice, it is often simpler to provide a homemade gluten-free lunch for your child to take to school.

The Individuals with Disabilities Education Act (IDEA)

The Individuals with Disabilities Education Act (IDEA) is a federal law that guarantees a free and appropriate education to all children who have disabilities that have an educational impact on their ability to learn at school. Specifically, it applies to children who have been diagnosed with:

- mental retardation
- hearing impairments (including deafness)
- speech or language impairments
- visual impairments (including blindness)
- serious emotional disturbance

- orthopedic impairments
- autism
- traumatic brain injury
- other health impairments (including epilepsy, diabetes, and attention deficit disorders)
- specific learning disabilities.

As mentioned above, the law does *not* apply to children who only have celiac disease, but does apply to children who have celiac disease in addition to one of the qualifying disabilities above.

Children who qualify under IDEA receive an Individualized Education Program (IEP). For children three and older, the IEP is a written plan that describes long-term goals and short-term objectives for learning, as well as the services that will be provided to help the child reach those goals, and the setting where the services will be provided. An IEP is developed by a team consisting of school personnel, parents, and the child himself, if he chooses to participate.

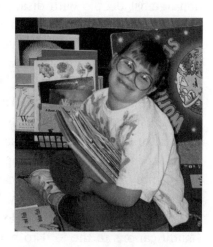

It is beyond the scope of this book to explain the basics of qualifying for services under IDEA, or to go into detail about writing good IEPs. You should know, however, that if your child has an IEP because he has Down syndrome, autism, or another disability, the IEP can include goals and services related to helping him learn to manage his celiac disease.

Remember, your child's IEP will be *individualized* to his needs and abilities, so it is impossible to list goals that would be appropriate for all children who have celiac disease in addition to another disability. Here are a few examples, though, that might be appropriate for some children:

- If the class as a whole has a unit on nutrition, a goal for your child might be to understand how gluten fits into the food pyramid, and what gluten-free substitutions can be made for foods listed on the pyramid.
- If your child is receiving speech therapy as a related service, a goal might be for him to learn to request gluten-free items in the cafeteria, either verbally or by using some kind of alternative and augmentative system (pictures of "safe" foods on a key ring, voice output computer, etc.).
- For an older child learning functional skills, goals could be related to learning to read and use a list of "safe" foods and ingredients when shopping or preparing foods.

- A child who continually tries to eat his classmates' (gluten-containing) food in the cafeteria or during school parties could have a plan for positive behavioral support in this area written into his IEP.

It is important to note that any student covered by IDEA is also covered by Section 504. He would therefore be able to obtain the same modifications to the school lunch program described above, as long as he had a doctor's prescription stating that need.

The Americans with Disabilities Act

The Americans with Disabilities Act (ADA) takes up where Section 504 of the Rehabilitation Act leaves off. Whereas Section 504 only prohibits discrimination against people with disabilities by agencies receiving federal funding, the ADA extends protections into many more areas of public life.

The ADA is divided into five titles or sections. For people with celiac disease, the sections with the most relevance are Title 1 (Employment) and Title III (Public Accommodations).

Title I: Employment. This section prohibits employers from discriminating against qualified individuals with disabilities during the application or hiring process, or when determining salary, benefits, or other aspects of employment. It prohibits employers from asking whether an applicant has a disability and refusing to hire someone solely because they have a disability, or because they are perceived as having a disability. If an employee tells his employer about his disability, however, then the employer must provide "reasonable accommodations" (modifications to the job) to help the employee succeed—provided the accommodation does not impose an "undue hardship" on the employer.

Title III: Public Accommodations. A public accommodation is a business, program, or agency that provides services or goods to the public. The ADA lists twelve categories of public accommodations, including: places of lodging (inns, hotels, motels); establishments serving food or drink; places of exhibition or entertainment (movie theaters, stadiums, concert halls); sales or retail establishments (stores of all kinds, shopping centers); places of public display or collection (museums, libraries); schools serving students of all ages; places of exercise or recreation (gyms, health spas, bowling alleys); places that provide testing services. *(Facilities run by religious entities and private clubs are excepted.)*

Under ADA, individuals with disabilities are entitled to "full and equal enjoyment of the goods, services, facilities, privileges, advantages, or accommodations" of any place of public accommodation.

For your child, this section of the ADA means that he should not be denied the opportunity to go anywhere or do anything because of his celiac disease.

For example, a child-care center may be required to change its policy regarding sharing foods, or a summer camp may need to make gluten-free menu items available as a way of accommodating your child's special diet. Likewise, it is against the law for a restaurant to refuse to serve people who require special diets due to a disability.

Who Is Covered by the ADA?

The ADA defines "disability" very broadly. Under this law, an individual is protected from discrimination if:

- He is perceived as having a disability. For instance, you and your child may not consider celiac disease the least bit disabling, but if an employer or other individual discriminates against your child because *he* thinks celiac disease is a disability, your child would be covered by the law.
- He is related to, or associated with, someone who has a disability. For example, it would be against the law for an employer to refuse to hire or promote you solely because he thinks you are the parent of a child with a disability, and that your child-care duties might be too time consuming.
- He actually has a disability that substantially limits a major life activity— caring for himself, performing manual tasks, walking, seeing, hearing, speaking, breathing, learning, working, thinking, concentrating, and interacting with other people.

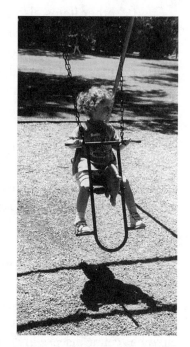

In reality, most families of children with celiac disease will likely never need to use the ADA to obtain the accommodations their child needs. Most restaurants are more than happy to serve people who need gluten-free meals; the vast majority of daycare centers, schools, and recreation departments will willingly work with you to handle your child's special dietary needs; and few employers would even dream of discriminating against an employee because he has celiac disease. However, on the off chance that you encounter someone who does perceive celiac disease as a disability worthy of discrimination, it is good to know that the ADA protects your child.

If you believe your child has been discriminated against under Titles I or III of the ADA, you can send a letter of complaint to The U.S. Department of Justice, Civil Rights Division, Coordination and Review Section. (See the Resource Guide for the address.) You may also bring a lawsuit against any business or program that you feel has discriminated against you or your child under ADA.

Income Tax Deductions

Considering what it can cost to keep your child on a gluten-free diet, it would be nice if you could write some of the extra cost off, wouldn't it? In fact, the Internal Revenue Service does allow income tax deductions for people with dietary restrictions. According to the Celiac Disease Foundation, there are four areas that qualify.

1. The law says that the *additional* expense of special dietary products may be deducted. For instance, if a "regular" loaf of bread costs $2.50 and a gluten-free loaf of bread costs $4.50, the $2.00 difference may be deducted. Special gluten-free mixes, pastas, and any other items also qualify.

2. The full cost of special items needed for a gluten-free diet may be deducted. The cost of xanthan gum (methyl cellulose), for instance, may be deducted, because it is used in gluten-free home-baked items, but is completely different from anything used in an ordinary recipe.

3. If you make a special trip to a specialty store to purchase gluten-free foods, the actual cost of your transportation to and from the store is deductible. If you are using your vehicle for the trip, you will need to check with the IRS for current mileage deduction amounts.

4. The full cost of postage or other delivery expenses on gluten-free purchases made by mail order are deductible.

The total amount of your deduction for gluten-free foods should be added to your other medical expenses that are reported on line 1 of Schedule A on Form 1040 (for taxpayers who itemize deductions).

If you are audited, you will need a letter from your doctor stating that your child has celiac disease and must adhere to a gluten-free diet for life. You will also need substantiation in the form of receipts, cash register tapes, or canceled checks for your gluten-free purchases, and a schedule showing how you computed your deductions for the gluten-free foods.

Appendix

Quick Start Diet Guide for Celiac Disease

Here is a quick and simple overview of the gluten-free (GF) diet. Not all areas of the diet are as clear-cut as portrayed by this Guide. This is intended to be used as a safe and temporary survival tool until the newly diagnosed celiac can gather additional information. Understanding these *dietary requirements* will enable you to read labels of food products and determine if a product is GF, not GF, or questionable. Questionable ingredients are those that do not give enough information to determine whether or not it is gluten free. Examples of these are modified food starch (the type of starch needs to be identified).

Celiac Disease (CD) is a chronic digestive disorder found in individuals who are genetically susceptible. Damage to the small intestine is caused by an immunologically toxic reaction to the ingestion of gluten. This does not allow food to be properly absorbed. Even small amounts of gluten in foods may affect those with celiac disease and result in health problems. Damage can occur to the small bowel even in the absence of symptoms.

Gluten is the generic name for certain types of proteins contained in the common cereal grains wheat, barley, rye, and oats and derivatives from these.

Allowed or Not Allowed?
Allowed
- Rice
- Corn
- Soy
- Potato
- Tapioca
- Bean
- Sorghum
- Quinoa
- Millet
- Buckwheat
- Arrowroot

- Amaranth
- Tef
- Nut flours

Not Allowed

The following grains contain **Gluten** and are **NOT ALLOWED in any form:**
- Wheat (durum, semolina, kamut, spelt)
- Rye
- Barley
- Oats
- Triticale

Frequently overlooked foods that often contain gluten:

- Breading
- Broth
- Coating mixes
- Communion wafers
- Croutons
- Imitation bacon
- Imitation seafood
- Marinades
- Pastas
- Processed meats
- Roux
- Sauces
- Self-basting poultry
- Soup bases
- Stuffings
- Thickeners

Wheat Free is not Gluten Free!

Wheat-free products may still contain rye, oats, barley, or ingredients that are not GF.

Labels

The key to understanding the GF diet is to become a good ingredient label reader. Food labels containing the following ingredients are **questionable** and **should not** be consumed **unless** you can **verify** they do not contain or are derived from prohibited grains:
- Brown rice syrup (frequently made from barley)
- Caramel color
- Dextrin (usually corn, but may be derived from wheat)

- Flour or cereal products
- Hydrolyzed vegetable protein (HVP), vegetable protein, hydrolyzed plant protein
- (HPP), or textured vegetable protein (TVP)
- Malt or malt flavoring (usually made from barley.) Okay if made from corn
- Malt vinegar
- Modified food starch or modified starch from unspecified or forbidden source
- Mono- & diglycerides (in dry products only)
- Flavorings in meat products
- Soy sauce or soy sauce solids (many soy sauces contain wheat)
- Vegetable gum

Clear Labels Are Safest

A clear label has no gluten-containing or questionable ingredients. If it has questionable ingredients, **avoid it** and find a comparable product that is GF. *Labels must be read every time you purchase food.* Some products remain GF for years, while others do not. You may verify ingredients by calling or writing a food manufacturer and specifying the ingredient and the lot number of the food in question. State your needs clearly—be patient, persistent, and polite.

If in doubt go without!

If unable to verify ingredients or the ingredient list is unavailable—**DO NOT EAT IT.** It is not worth triggering your immune system and the damage to the small intestine that occurs every time gluten is consumed, regardless of the amount eaten, or whether symptons are present.

One new food at a time

When adding a new food item to your diet, particularly one that has questionable ingredients that you have cleared, introduce only one new food at a time. Listen to your body for adverse reactions before starting a second new food item.

Contamination
Food Preparation

When preparing gluten-free foods they must not come into contact with food containing gluten. Contamination can occur if foods are prepared on common surfaces, or with utensils that are not thoroughly cleaned after preparing gluten-containing foods. Using a common toaster for GF bread and regular bread is a major source of contamination. Flour sifters should not be shared with gluten-containing flours. Deep fried foods cooked in oil shared with breaded products should not be consumed. Spreadable condiments in containers shared by others may also provide contamination. When a knife is dipped into a condiment for a second time, the condiment becomes contaminated with crumbs (i.e., mustard, mayonnaise, jam, peanut butter, and margarine).

Resource Guide

People and Places You Should Know About

Information, contacts, and references for celiac disease are changing by the second. Please forgive any information that is not current, or any listings that have unintentionally been overlooked; all reference information included in this book is current at the time of printing.

Also note that suppliers, manufacturers, distributors, and stores mentioned do not necessarily carry gluten-free products. Their contact information is provided so that the reader may easily contact the company to verify status of products.

Organizations
National Organizations and Support Groups

Many of these organizations have local chapters; contact the national support group to obtain contact information. Most organizations also offer free or low-cost pamphlets, fact sheets, or other publications, or make their publications available free of charge online.

American Autoimmune Related
  Diseases Association
22100 Gratiot Avenue
Detroit, MI 48021
(810) 776-3900; (810) 776-3903 (Fax)
aarda@aol.com
www.aarda.org

American Celiac Society
  National Headquarters
5p Crystal Ave.
West Orange, NJ 07052-4114
Contact: Annette Bentley (973) 325-8837
amerceliacsoc@netscape.net

American Dietetic Association
216 W. Jackson Blvd.
Chicago, IL 60606-6995
(312) 899-0040; (800) 366-1655;
(312) 899-4899 (Fax)
hotline@eatright.org
www.eatright.org

Celiac Disease Foundation (CDF)
13251 Ventura Blvd., Suite 1
Studio City, CA 91604-1838
(818) 990-2354; (818) 990-2379 (Fax)
cdf@celiac.org
www.celiac.org

Celiac Sprue Association (CSA/USA)
P.O. Box 31700
Omaha, NE 68131-0700
(402) 558-0600; (402) 558-1347 (Fax)
celiacs@csaceliacs.org
www.csaceliacs.org

Food Allergy Network (FAN)
10400 Eaton Place, Suite107
Fairfax, VA 22030
(800) 929-4040; (703) 691-2713 (Fax)
fan@worldweb.net
www.foodallergy.org

Gluten Intolerance Group of North America (GIG)
15110 10th Avenue S.W., Suite A
Seattle, WA 98166-1820
(206) 246-6652; (206) 246-6531 (Fax)
info@gluten.net
www.gluten.net

Office of the Americans with Disabilities Act
Public Access Section
Civil Rights Division
U.S. Department of Justice
P.O. Box 66738
Washington, DC 20035-6738
(800) 514-0301; (800) 514-0383 (TDD)
www.usdoj.gov/crt/ada/adahom1.htm

Office of Special Education Programs (OSEP)
Mary E. Switzer Building, Room 3006
330 C Street, S.W.
Washington, DC 20202
(202) 205-5465
www.ed.gov/offices/OSERS/OSEP/index.html

U.S. Department of Agriculture
Food and Nutrition Service
3101 Park Center Drive, Room 819
Alexandria, VA 22302
(703) 305-2286
webmaster@fns.usda.gov
www.fns.usda.gov/fns

U.S. Department of Education
Office for Civil Rights
Customer Service Team
Mary E. Switzer Building, Room 5000
330 C Street, S.W.
Washington, DC 20202
(202) 205-5413; (800) 421-3481;
(877) 521-2172 (TTY); (202) 205-9862 (Fax)
OCR@ED.Gov
www.ed.gov/offices/OCR

International Organizations and Support Groups

Canadian Celiac Association (CCA)
190 Britannia Road East, Unit #11
Mississauga, Ontario, Canada L4Z 1W6
(905) 507-6208; (800) 363-7296;
(905) 507-4673 (Fax)
www.celiac.ca; www.celiac.edmonton.ab.ca;
www.penny.ca/Hamilton.htm

Coeliac Society of Australia
11 Barlyn Road, Mount Waverley, 3149
P.O. Box 89, Holmesglen, 3148
(03) 9808-5566; (03) 9808-9922 (Fax)
www.coeliac.org.au

Coeliac Society of New Zealand
27 Tuna Terrace
Titahi Bay, New Zealand
(03) 479-3744; (64 3) 479-7344
phil.sheard@STONEBOW.OTAGO.AC.NZ

Coeliac Society of the United Kingdom
P.O. Box 220
High Wycome, Bucks HP 11 2HY
England, UK
(44) 494-437278; (44) 494-474349 (Fax)
www.coeliac.co.uk

Deutsche Zoeliakie-Gesellschaft (German
  Celiac Society)
Filderhauptstrasse 61
D-70599 Stuttgart 70, Germany
(49) 07-11-45-45-14; (49) 07-11-4567817 (Fax)
info@dzg-online.de
http://home.t-online.de/home/DZG.E.V./
  homepage.htm

Other Organizations and Support Groups

Celiac Disease On-Line Support Group
  (Chat Room)
Operator and Chat Moderator: Abigail Neuman
www.delphi.com/celiac

Celiac Kids' Club (Westchester Celiac Sprue
  Support Group)
Contact: Marisa Frederick
264 Scotchtown Road
Goshen, NY 10924
(845) 294-1385
CeliacWestchNY@aol.com

Celiac Support Group for Children
11 Level Acres Road
Attleboro, MA 02703
(508) 399-6229; (508) 399-6685 (Fax)
csgc@ix.netcom.com
www.members.home.net/kellyleech/celiac/
  csgc.html

Celiac Support Page
postmaster@celiac.com
www.celiac.com

Gluten Free Casein Free (GFCF) Diet Support
  Group
P.O. Box 1692
Palm Harbor, FL 34682
comments@gfctdiet.com
www.gfcfdiet.com

Research Organizations

Children's Hospital, Los Angeles
Center for Celiac Research
Contact: Christine Rongley
4650 Sunset Blvd.
MS #78-Division of Gastroenterology
Los Angeles, CA 90027
(323) 669-2181; (323) 664-0718 (Fax)
http://chla.org/gastroenterology.cfm

The Columbia Genome Center
Columbia University College of Physicians
  and Surgeons
Celiac Disease Center
161 Fort Washington Avenue, Room 645
New York, NY 10032
(212) 305-5590; (212) 305-3738
www.columbia.edu

Mayo Clinic
Dr. Joseph Murray
200 First Street S.W.
Rochester, MN 55905
(507) 284-2511; (800) 291-1128;
(507) 284-0161 (Fax)
www.mayohealth.org; www.mayoclinic.com

University of Utah
391 Chipeta Way, Suite D
Salt Lake City, UT 84108
(801) 581-5075; (800) 444-8638 ex.15075
erin@episun5.med.utah.edu

University of California, San Diego (UCSD)
Celiac Disease Clinic
Martin Kagnoff, M.D.
9500 Gilman Dr.
La Jolla, CA 92093
(858) 534-4622
Immunology@ucsd.edu
http://medicine.ucsd.edu/mucosalimmunology

University of Maryland
Center for Celiac Research (CFCR)
Alessio Fasano, M.D. and Karoly Horvath, M.D.
700 West Lombard Street
Baltimore, MD 21201
(410) 706-2715
www.celiaccenter.org

Friends of Celiac Disease Research, Inc.
8832 North Port Washington Road, # 204
Milwaukee, WI 53217
(414) 540-6679; (414) 540-0587 (Fax)
friends@aero.net
www.friendsofceliac.com
  (devoted to *funding* research and education)

Testing Laboratories

EnteroLab
email@enterolab.com
www.enterolab.com

IMMCO Diagnostics, Inc.
60 Pine View Drive
Amherst, NY 14228
(800) 537-TEST; (716) 691-0466
IMMTEST@aol.com
www.immcodiagnostics.com

Labspec
Gluten Enteropathy/Coeliac Support Group
73 Old Mill Way
Durban North, South Africa 4051
(031) 5633109
lucoll@mweb.co.za
www.labspec.co.za

Prometheus GI Disease Management
5739 Pacific Center Blvd.
San Diego, CA 92121
(858) 824-0895; (888) 423-5227;
(858) 824-0896 (Fax)
email@prometheus-labs.com
www.prometheus-labs.com

Specialty Laboratories
2211 Michigan Ave.
Santa Monica, CA 90404-3900
(310) 828-6543; (800) 421-7110;
(310) 828-6634 (Fax)
speciality@specialtylabs.com
www.specialtylabs.com

Sources of Medical and Nutritional Reference Information

American Journal of Clinical Nutrition
9650 Rockville Pike, L-2310
Bethesda, MD 20814-3998
(301) 530-7038; (301) 571-5728 (Fax)
www.ajcn.org

Autism and Diet Website
www.advimoss.no/GFCF_results.htm

Better Health USA
1620 W. Oakland Park Blvd., Suite 401
Ft. Lauderdale, FL 33311
(800) 684-2231; (954) 739-2780 (Fax)
info@betterhealthusa.com
www.betterhealthusa.com

Down Syndrome: Health Issues
www.ds-health.com/celiac.htm

An Experimental Intervention for Autism:
    Understanding and Implementing a Gluten
    and Casein Free Diet
Lisa S. Lewis, Ph.D.
156 E. Delaware Avenue
Pennington, NJ 08534
lisas156@aol.com
www.princeton.edu/~serge/ll/gfpak.html

Finer Health and Nutrition
Kenneth Fine, M.D.
email@finerhealth.com
www.finerhealth.com

Healthfinder
A Service of the U.S. Department of Health and
    Human Services
200 Independence Avenue, S.W.
Washington, DC 20201
(202) 619-0257; (877) 696-6775
healthfinder@health.org
www.healthfinder.gov

Healthgate
(800) 434-GATE
support@healthgate.com
www.healthgate.com

Medscape, Inc.
20500 N.W. Evergreen Parkway
Hillsboro, OR 97124
(503) 531-7000; (503) 531-7001 (Fax)
www.medscape.com

The Merck Manual
Merck & Co., Inc.
One Merck Drive
P.O. Box 100
Whitehouse Station, NJ 08889-0100
(800) 819-9546; (732) 594-1187 (Fax)
www.merck.com

National Digestive Diseases Clearing House
    (NDDIC)
A Service of National Institute of Diabetes &
    Digestive & Kidney Diseases (NIDDK-NIH)
2 Information Way
Bethesda, MD 20892-3570
(301) 654-3810
nddic@info.niddk.nih.gov
www.niddk.nih.gov

National Health Information Center (NHIC)
P.O. Box 1133
Washington, DC 20013-1133
(800) 336-4797; (301)565-4167;
(301) 984-4256 (Fax)
nhicinfo@health.org
www.nhic.org

National Organization for Rare Disorders, Inc.
(NORD)
P.O. Box 8923
New Fairfield, CT 06812-8923
(203) 746-6518; (800) 999-6673
(203) 746-6481 (Fax)
orphan@rarediseases.org
www.rarediseases.org

Nutribase Directory of Food and Supplement
Manufacturers
info@nutribase.com
www.nutribase.com/dfm.htm

Sprue Nik Press Medical/Research Articles
Index
34638 Beechwood
Farmington, MI 48335
(248) 926-1228
www.enabling.org/ia/celiac/sn/spinmed.html

United States National Library of Medicine
(NLM)
8600 Rockville Pike
Bethesda, MD 20894
(888) FINDNLM
custserv@nlm.nih.gov
www.nlm.nih.gov

Listservs

A listserv is an Internet "mailing list" which allows participants to post questions, answers, and comments on a list that is distributed by e-mail to all participants.

Autistic Kids on a Gluten-Free Diet Listserv
To subscribe: Visit www.onelist.com and
subscribe to the list called "gfcfkids."

Celiac Listserv
To subscribe: Send e-mail to
Listserv@maelstrom.stjohns.edu with "subscribe
celiac" in subject heading (be sure to send this
e-mail from the address you want your listserv
e-mails sent to).

Celiac Listserv—Cel-Kids News Group
To subscribe: Send e-mail to
Listserv@maelstrom.stjohns.edu with "subscribe
cel-kids" in subject heading (be sure to send this
e-mail from the address you want your listserv
e-mails sent to).

Website Collections/Links

Celiac Information
Listowners:
Bill Elkus, maxwell@lamg.com
Michael Jones, mjones@digital.net
Jim Lyles, lyles@tir.com
www.enabling.org/ia/celiac

Database of Gluten-Free Manufacturers
Operator: Linda Blanchard
linda@ccgs.com
www.nowheat.com

Gluten-Free Links
Operator: Don Wiss
donwiss@panix.com
www.gflinks.com

The Kitchen Link: Wheat Free and Gluten Free
   Recipes and Resources
help@kitchenlink.com
www.kitchenlink.com/wheatfree.html

Nutribase Directory of Food and Supplement
   Manufacturers
info@nutribase.com
www.nutribase.com/dfm.htm

Activities and Camps for Children with Celiac Disease

Camp Celiac for Kids
Celiac Support Group for Children
11 Level Acres Road
Attleboro, MA 02703
(508) 399-6229; 508-399-6685 (Fax)
csgc@ix.netcom.com
www.members.home.net/kellyleech/celiac/
csgc.html

GIG Kid's Camp
Gluten Intolerance Group
15110 10th Ave S.W., Suite A
Seattle, WA 98166-1820
(206) 246-6652; (206) 246-6531
info@gluten.net
www.gluten.net

Shopping
Guides to Gluten-Free Shopping

The Celiac Database
Operator: Chuck Brandt
P.O. Box 5605
Wilmington, DE 19808-0605
(302) 999-1144; (302) 999-9794 (Fax)
info@celiacdatabase.org
http://www.celiacdatabase.org

Erewhon Natural Foods Market
Celiac Shopping Guide
shop@erewhonmarket.com
www.erewhonmarket.com/
celiacshoppingguide.html

Gluten Free Food List
Operator: Abigail Neuman
www.geocities.com/HotSprings/Spa/4003/gf-
index.html

Gluten-Free Food Vendor Directory
Operator: Don Wiss
donwiss@panix.com
www.gfmall.com

Gluten-Free InfoWeb
2422 Fox Hollow Drive
Pittsburgh, PA 15237
CeliacInfo@aol.com
http://www.glutenfreeinfo.com

Gluten-Free Pocket Guides and Databases for
    Food/Drugs
Operator: Clan Thompson
951 Main Street
Stoneham, ME 04231
(207) 928-3303
observer@nxi.com
www.clanthompson.com

Mail-Order and Online Sources of Gluten-Free Products

Cecilia's Gluten-Free Grocery
PMB 171
3702 S. Virginia Street G12
Reno, NV 89502-7510
(775) 827-0672; (800) 491-2760;
(775) 827-5850 (Fax)
info@glutenfreegrocery.com
www.glutenfreegrocery.com

DeRoMa (Glutino Brand)
1118 Rue Berlier
Laval, Quebec, Canada H7L 3R9
(450) 629-7689; (800) 363-DIET
info@glutino.com
www.glutino.com

Ener-G Foods
P.O. Box 84487
Seattle, WA 98124-5787
(800) 331-5222; (206) 764-3398
heidi@ener-g.com
www.ener-g.com

Frankferd Foods
www.frankferd.com

Gluten-Free Cookie Jar
P.O. Box 52
Trevose, PA 19053
(215) 355-9403; (888) GLUTEN-0;
(215) 355-7991 (Fax)
glutenfreecookiejar@yahoo.com
www.glutenfreecookiejar.com

Gluten Free Delights
P.O. Box 284
Cedar Falls, IA 50613
(319) 266-7167; (888) 403-1806;
(319) 268-7355 (Fax)
ZEJG11A@prodigy.com
www.glutenfreedelights.com

Gluten-Free Mall
info@glutenfreemall.com
www.glutenfreemall.com

Gluten Free Pantry
P.O. Box 840
Glastonbury, CT 06033
(860) 633-3826; (800) 291-8386;
(860) 633-6853 (Fax)
pantry@glutenfree.com
www.glutenfree.com

The Gluten-Free Trading Company
604A W. Lincoln Avenue
Milwaukee, WI 53215
(414) 385-9950; (888) 993-9933;
(414) 385-9915 (Fax)
info@gluten-free.net
www.gluten-free.net

Gluten Solutions, Inc.
737 Manhattan Blvd., Ste. B
Manhattan Beach, CA 90266
(310) 939-7559; (888) 8-GLUTEN
info@glutensolutions.com
www.glutensolutions.com

Glutino
See DeRoMa

Kinnikinick Foods
10306-112 Street
Edmonton, Alberta, Canada
T5K 1N1
(780) 424-2900; (877) 503-4466;
(780) 421-0456 (Fax)
info@kinnikinnick.com
www.kinnikinnick.com

Menu Direct Corporation—Dietary Specialties
865 Centennial Ave.
Piscataway, NJ 08854
(888) MENU 123; (732) 980-6770 (Fax)
webinfo@menudirect.com
www.dietspec.com

Miss Roben's
P.O. Box 1149
Frederick, MD 21702
(301) 665-9580; (800) 891-0083;
(301) 665-9584 (Fax)
info@missroben.com
www.missroben.com

Really Great Food Co.
P.O. Box 2239
St. James, NY 11780
(800) 593-5377; (631) 361-6920 (Fax)
chris@reallygreatfood.com
www.reallygreatfood.com

Schär
Dr. Schär GmbH
Winkelau 5
I-39014 Postal (BZ)
(+39) 0473-293300
info@schaer.com
www.schaer.com/p5100uk.html

Sylvan Border Farm Gluten-Free Products
Mendocino Gluten-Free Products, Inc.
P.O. Box 277
Willits, CA 95490
(800) 297-5399; (707) 459-1834 (Fax)
http://catalog.com/mendo/gcm/sylvan.html

Manufacturers and Retailers

Contact information for supermarket chains, manufacturers, and other distributors of food and other products is provided below so you can check the gluten-free status of particular products.

Albertson's (supermarkets)
250 Parkcenter Blvd.
Boise, ID 83706
(888) 746-7252; (208) 395-3302 (Fax)
cs_online@albertsons/com
www.albertsons.com

Alpineaire Foods
4031 Alvis Ct.
Rocklin, CA 95677
(800) 322-6325; (916) 824-5020 (Fax)
www.gluten-freecafe.com

Amy's Kitchen
P.O. Box 7868
Santa Rosa, CA 95407
(707) 578-7188; (707) 570-0306

Annie's Naturals
792 Foster Hill Rd.
North Calais, VT 05650
(802) 456-8866; (800) 434-1234;
(802) 456-8865 (Fax)
info@anniesnaturals.com
www.anniesnaturals.com

Arrowhead Mills
P.O. Box 2059
Hereford, TX 79045
(800) 749-0730; (806) 364-8242 (Fax)

Aurora Foods
1000 St. Louis Union Station
St. Louis, MO 63103
(314) 241-0303; (888) 349-1998;
(314) 613-5567 (Fax)
www.aurorafoods.com

Authentic Foods
1850 W. 169th St., Ste. B
Gardena, CA 90247
(800) 806-4737; (310) 366-7612;
(310) 366-6938 (Fax)
sales@authenticfoods.com
www.authenticfoods.com

Balance Bars
1015 Mark Ave.
Carpinteria, CA 93013
(800) 678-4246; (805) 566-0235 (Fax)
healthy@balance.com
www.balance.com

Beatrice Group
770 N. Springdale Rd.
Waukesha, WI 53186
(262) 782-2750; (800) 227-6202
www.beatricefoods.com

Ben & Jerry's Homemade, Inc.
30 Community Drive
South Burlington, VT 05403-6828
(802) 846-1500; (800) 726-6748
www.benandjerrys.com

Best Foods
International Plaza
700 Sylvan Avenue
Englewood Cliffs, NJ 07632-9976
(201) 894-4000; (800) 338-8831
www.bestfoods.com

Betty Crocker (Signature Brands/General Mills)
P.O. Box 279
Ocala, FL 34478-0279
(800) 328-8360; (800) 456-9573;
(800) 328-1144; (352) 402-9451 (Fax)
www.bettycrocker.com

Blue Diamond Growers
1802 C Street
Sacramento, CA 95814
(916) 442-0771; (800) 987-2329
customerservice@bluediamondgrowers.com
www.bluediamondnuts.com

Cabot Creamery Cooperative
Main Street
Cabot, VT 05647
(188) TRY-CABOT
info@cabotcheese.com
www.cabotcheese.com

Cadbury/Shweppes
25 Berkeley Square
London, England
W1X6HT
www.cadbury.co.uk

Campbell's Soup Company
Campbell Place
Camden, NJ 08103-1701
(800) 257-8443; (800) 410-7687
www.campbellssoup.com

'Cause You're Special Co.
P.O. Box 316
Phillips, WI 54555
(815) 877-6722; (603) 754-0245 (Fax)
questions@causeyourespecial.com
www.causeyourespecial.com

Cecilia's Gluten-Free Grocery
PMB 171
3702 S Virginia Street G12
Reno, NV 89502-7510
(775) 827-0672; (800) 491-2760
(775) 827-5850 (Fax)
info@glutenfreegrocery.com,
www.glutenfreegrocery.com

Celestial Seasonings Tea
4600 Sleepy Time Drive
Boulder, CO 80301
(800) 351-8175; (303) 581-1294 (Fax)
www.celestialseasonings.com

Chebe Bread (Prima Provisions)
P.O. Box 27085
West Des Moines, IA 50266
(515) 223-5007; (800) 217-9510
info@chebe.com
www.chebe.com

Chicken of the Sea International
Consumer Affairs
P.O. Box 85568
San Diego, CA 92138-5568
www.chickenofthesea.com

Classico
International Gourmet Specialties Company
10 E. Broad Street
Columbus, OH 43215-3799
(800) 727-8260
www.classico.com

Coca Cola
Industry and Consumer Affairs
P.O. Drawer 1734
Atlanta, GA
30301
(800) GET-COKE
www.cocacola.com

Coldstone Creamery
16101 N. 82nd Street, #A4
Scottsdale, AZ 85260
(480) 348-1704; (480) 348-1718 (Fax)
www.coldstonecreamery.com

Colgate-Palmolive
(800) 338-8388; (800) 468-6502
www.colgate.com

Costco (Price Club)
P.O. Box 34331
Issaquah, WA 98027
(800) 774-2678
www.costco.com

Creative Rice Baking
P.O. Box 6281
Rock Island, IL 61204
creativericebaking@revealed.net
http://home.revealed.net/creativericebaking

Dannon
Dannon Consumer Response Center
P.O. Box 90296
Allentown, PA 18109-0296
(800) 321-2174; (877) DANNONUS
www.dannon.com

Delimex
7878 Airway Road
San Diego, CA 92154
(800) DELIMEX; (619) 671-0600 (Fax)
gpanzari@delimex.com
www.delimex.com

DeRoMa (Glutino Brand)
1118 Rue Berlier
Laval, Quebec, Canada H7L 3R9
(450) 629-7689; (800) 363-DIET
info@glutino.com
www.glutino.com

Dreyer's
5929 College Avenue
Oakland, CA 94618
(877) 437-3937
www.dreyers.com

Duncan Hines
1000 St. Louis Station, Suite 300
St. Louis, MO 63103
(800) 845-7286
www.duncanhines.com

Edy's Ice Cream
5929 College Avenue
Oakland, CA 94618
(800) 777-3397
www.edys.com

Ener-G Foods
P.O. Box 84487
Seattle, WA 98124-5787
(800) 331-5222; (206) 764-3398
www.ener-g.com

Epicurean International, Inc. (Thai Kitchen)
P.O. Box 13242
Berkeley, CA 94701
(510) 268-0209; (800) 967-8424
(510) 834-3102 (Fax)
info@thaikitchen.com
www.thaikitchen.com

Fantastic Foods
1250 N. McDowell Blvd.
Petaluma, CA
94954
(707) 778-7607; (800) 888-7801
(707) 778-7607 (Fax)
AskUs@fantasticfoods.com
www.fantasticfoods.com

Farley's (Nabisco)
2945 W. 31st Street
Chicago, IL 60623
(312) 254-0900; (800) 541-1222
(312) 254-0795 (Fax)
www.nabisco.com

Farmer John
Clougherty Packing Company
3049 E. Vernon Avenue
Los Angeles, CA 90058
(323) 583-4621; (800) 432-7637
(323) 584-1699 (Fax)
farmerjohn@farmerjohn.com
www.farmerjohn.com

Favorite Brands International (Nabisco)
Nabisco Consumer Affairs
100 DeForest Avenue
P.O. Box 1911
East Hanover, NJ 07936-1911
(800) 244-4596
www.nabisco.com

Fisher Nuts
John B. Sanfilippo & Son, Inc.
2299 Busse Road
Elk Grove Village, IL 60007-6057
(847) 593-2300; (847) 593-3085 (Fax)
www.fishernuts.com

Fleischmann's
See Beatrice Group, Inc.

Food For Life Baking Co., Inc.
2991 E. Doherty Street
Corona, CA 91719
(800) 797-5090; (888) 458-8360
(909) 279-1784 (Fax)
info@food-for-life.com
www.food-for-life.com

Frankferd Farms Foods
www.frankferd.com

Friendly Ice Cream Corporation
1855 Boston Road
Wilbraham, MA 01095
(800) 966-9970
www.friendly.com

Frito Lay
P.O. Box 660634
Dallas, TX 75266-0634
(800) 352-4477
www.fritolay.com

Frookie
2070 Maple Street
Des Plaines, IL 60018
(888) FROOKIE; (847)699-3201(Fax)
www.frookie.com

G! Foods
3536 17th Street
San Francisco, CA 94110
(415) 255-2139, (415) 863-3359 (Fax)
gfoods@SHELL12.BA.BEST.COM
www.g-foods.com

Genisoy Products Company
2351 N. Watney Way, Suite C
Fairfield, CA 94533
(707) 399-2510; (888) GENISOY
(707) 399-2518 (Fax)
sales@mloproducts.com
www.genisoy.com

Gifts of Nature
P.O. Box 309
Corvallis, MT 59828
(406) 961-1529
giftsofnature@netzero.com
www.giftsofnature.net

Gillian's Foods, Inc.
462 Proctor Avenue
Revere, MA 02151-5730
(781) 286-4095; (781) 286-1933 (Fax)
R357BOBO@aol.com
www.gilliansfoods.com

Glutano
Unit 270 Centennial Park, Centennial Avenue
Elstree, Borehamwood Herts
United Kingdom   WD6 3SS
(020) 8953-4444; (020) 8953-8285 (Fax)
info@glutenfree-foods.co.uk
www.glutenfree-foods.co.uk

Gluten-Free Cookie Jar
P.O. Box 52
Trevose, PA 19053
(215) 355-9403; (888) GLUTEN-0;
(215) 355-7991 (Fax)
questions@glutenfreecookiejar.com
www.glutenfreecookiejar.com

Gluten Free Delights
P.O. Box 284
Cedar Falls, IA 50613
(319) 266-7167; (888) 403-1806;
(319) 268-7355 (Fax)
ZEJG11A@prodigy.com
www.glutenfreedelights.com

Gluten-Free Mall
info@glutenfreemall.com
www.glutenfreemall.com

Gluten-Free Pantry
P.O. Box 840
Glastonbury, CT 06033
(860) 633-3826; (800) 291-8386;
(860) 633-6853 (Fax)
pantry@glutenfree.com
www.glutenfree.com

The Gluten-Free Trading Company
604A W. Lincoln Avenue
Milwaukee, WI 53215
(414) 385-9950; (888) 993-9933;
(414) 385-9915 (Fax)
info@gluten-free.net
www.gluten-free.net

Gluten Solutions, Inc.
737 Manhattan Blvd., Ste. B
Manhattan Beach, CA 90266
(310) 939-7559; (888) 8-GLUTEN
info@glutensolutions.com
www.glutensolutions.com

Glutino
See DeRoMa

Haagen-Dazs
Glen Pointe Center East
Teaneck, NJ 07666
(800) 767-0120
www.haagendazs.com

Health Valley
16100 Foothill Blvd.
Irwindale, CA 91706-7811
(800) 423-4846
www.healthvalley.com

Heinz U.S.A.
P.O. Box 57
Pittsburgh, PA 15230
(800) 872-2229; (800) 255-5750
(800) 568-8602 (Fax)
www.heinz.com

Herb-Ox
See Hormel

Hershey's
P.O. Box 815
Hershey, PA 17033-0815
(800) 468-1714
www.hersheys.com

Hidden Valley
Oakland, CA 94612
(800) 53-SAUCE
www.hiddenvalley.com

Hillshire Farm & Kahn's
P.O. Box 25111
Cincinnati, OH 45225
(800) 328-2426
www.hillshirefarm.com

Hol-Grain
www.holgrain.com

Hormel
P.O. Box 800
Austin, MN 55912
(800) 523-4635
www.hormel.com

Hunt-Wesson Inc.
P.O. Box 4800
Fullerton, CA 92634-4800
(800) 633-0112; (800) 457-6649
www.hunt-wesson.com

Imagine Foods, Inc.
350 Cambridge Avenue, #350
Palo Alto, CA 94306
(415) 327-1444; (800) 333-6339;
(415) 327-1459 (Fax)
www.imaginefoods.com

Jet-Puffed Marshmallows (Nabisco)
100 DeForest Avenue
P.O. Box 1911
East Hanover, NJ 07936-1911
(800) 244-4596
www.jetpuffed.com

Jimmy Dean Foods
8000 Centerview Parkway, Suite 400
Cordova, TN 38018
(800) 925-DEAN
www.jimmydean.com

Just Born
1300 Stefko Blvd.
Bethlehem, PA 18016
(800) 445-5787; (800) 543-4981 (Fax)
www.justborn.com

Kelloggs
Consumer Affairs
1 Kellogg Square
Battle Creek, MI 49016-1986
(800) 962-1413
www.kelloggs.com

Kelloggs (UK)
www.kelloggs.co.uk

Kingsmill Foods Co. LTD
(416) 755-1124; (800) 737-7976
www.kingsmillfoods.com

Kinnikinnick Foods
10306-112 Street
Edmonton, Alberta, Canada
T5K 1N1
(780) 424-2900; (877) 503-4466;
(780) 421-0456 (Fax)
info@kinnikinnick.com
www.kinnikinnick.com

Kitchen Basics, Inc.
P.O. Box 41022
Brecksville, OH 44141
(440) 838-1344; (480) 998-8622
info@kitchenbasics.net
www.kitchenbasics.net

Kozy Shack
(516) 938-1200
www.kozyshack.com

Kraft General Foods, Inc.
Consumer Response and Information
Kraft Court
Glenview, IL 60025
(800) 323-0768; (800) 543-5335
www.kraftfoods.com

Land-O-Lakes
P.O. Box 64050
St. Paul, MN 55164-0050
(800) 328-4155; (651) 481-2959 (Fax)
www.landolakes.com/new

Lawry's Foods, Inc.
700 Palisade Avenue
Englewood Cliffs, NJ 07632
(800) 745-9232; (800) 9LAWRYS
www.lawrys.com

Lays Products
See Frito Lay

Lea & Perrins
(800) 987-4674; (800) 338-8831
lpinfo@leaperrinsus.danone.com
www.lea-and-perrins.com

Legumes Plus
N. 204 Fairweather Street
Fairfield, WA 99012
(800) 845-1349; (509) 283-2314 (Fax)
www.legumesplus.com

Lifesavers (Nabisco)
P.O. Box 41
Salem, OR 27102
(800) 541-1222
www.nabisco.com

Lipton
700 Palisade Avenue
Englewood Cliffs, NJ 07632
(800) 697-7887; (800) 697-7897
www.lipton.com

Lipton (Canada)
(800) 565-7273

Log Cabin
See Aurora Foods, Inc.

Louis Rich
P.O. Box 7188
Madison, WI 53707
(800) 722-1421
www.louisrich.com

M&M Mars
High Street
Hackettstown, NJ 07840
(908) 852-1000; (800) 222-0293
www.mars.com

McCormick & Co., Inc.
211 Schilling Circle
Hunt Valley, MD 21031
(800) 632-5847; (410) 527-6267 (Fax)
www.mccormick.com

Mahatma
c/o Riviana Foods Inc.
P.O. Box 2636
Houston, TX 77252
(800) 226-9522; (713) 942-1826 (Fax)
info@riviana.com
www.mahatmarice.com

Malt-O-Meal
701 W. 5th Street
Northfield, MN 55057-0180
(800) 753-3029
ca@malt-o-meal.com
www.malt-o-meal.com

Manischewitz Food Products Corp.
One Manischewitz Plaza
Jersey City, NY 07302
(201) 333-3700 (ask for Deborah Ross)
info@manischewitz.com
www.manischewitz.com

Menu Direct Corporation - Dietary Specialties
865 Centennial Avenue
Piscataway, NJ 08854
(888) MENU 123; (732) 980-6770 (Fax)
webinfo@menudirect.com
www.dietspec.com

Miss Roben's
P.O. Box 1149
Frederick, MD 21702
(301) 665-9580; (800) 891-0083;
(301) 665-9584 (Fax)
info@missroben.com
www.missroben.com

Motts USA
Stanford, CT 06905-0800
(800) 426-4891
www.motts.com

Mr. Spice
Lang Naturals
850 Aquidneck Avenue
Newport, RI 02842
(401) 848-7700); (800) SAUCE-IT;
(401) 848-7701 (Fax)
customerservice@MrSpice.com
www.mrspice.com

Mrs. Butterworth's
See Aurora Foods, Inc.
www.mrsbutterworths.com

Mrs. Leeper's Pasta
12455 Kerran Street, Suite 200
Poway, CA 92064-6855
(858) 486-1101; (858) 486-5115 (Fax)
mlpinc@pacbell.net
www.mrsleeperspasta.com

Nabisco Brands, Inc.
P.O. Box 1911
E. Hanover, NJ 07936
(800) 622-4726
www.nabisco.com

Nature's Hilights, Inc.
P.O. Box 3526
Chico, CA 95928
(916) 342-6154; (800) 313-6454;
(916) 342-3130 (Fax)
nhi@maxinet.com

Nature's Life
7180 Lampson Avenue
Garden Grove, CA
92841
(800) 854-6837; (714) 379-6501 (Fax)
info@natlife.com
www.natlife.com

Nelson David of Canada
Celimix Brand Gluten-Free Foods
101-193 Dumoulin Street
Winnipeg, Manitoba R2H 0E4
Canada
(204) 237-9161; (204) 231-2883 (Fax)
Information available at www.glutenfreemall.com

Nestlé
P.O. Box 39487
Salem, OR 44139-0487
(800) 441-2525; (800) 258-6728;
(800) 851-0512
www.nestle.com

Nestlé (Willy Wonka Division)
(800) 299-6652

Newman's Own Organics
P.O. Box 2098
Aptos, CA 95001
(408) 685-2866; (800) 444-8705
www.newmansownorganics.com

Ore-Ida Foods, Inc. (Heinz)
P.O. Box 10
Boise, ID
83707
(800) 892-2401
www.oreida.com

Oscar Mayer Foods Corporation
P.O. Box 7188
Madison, WI 53707
(800) 672-2710; (800) 222-2323
www.oscarmayer.com

Pacific Grain Products, Inc.
P.O. Box 2060
Woodland, CA 95776
(916) 662-5056; (800) 49-BEANS
(916) 662-6074 (Fax)
www.pacificgrain.com

Pamela's Products
335 Allerton Avenue
South San Francisco, CA 94080
(650) 952-4546; (650) 742-6643 (Fax)
info@pamelasproducts.com
www.pamelasproducts.com

Pastariso (Rice Innovations Inc.)
1773 Bayly Street
Pickering, Ontario, Canada
L1W2Y7
(905) 451-7423

Pepsi-Co Food Services
6606 LBJ Freeway, #150A
Dallas, TX 75240
(800) 433-2652
www.pepsi.com

Planter's (Nabisco)
Nabisco Consumer Affairs
100 DeForest Avenue
P.O. Box 1911
East Hanover, NJ 07936-1911
(800) 8NABNET
www.planters.com

The Quaker Oats Company
P.O. Box 049003
Chicago, IL 60604-9003
(312) 222-7707; (800) 234-6281;
(800) 856-5781
www.quakeroats.com

Quinoa Corp
P.O. Box 1039
Torrance, CA 90505
(310) 530-8666; (310) 530-8764 (Fax)
quinoacorp@aol.com
www.quinoa.net

Really Great Food Co.
P.O. Box 2239
St. James, NY 11780
(800) 593-5377; (631) 361-6920 (Fax)
chris@reallygreatfood.com
www.reallygreatfood.com

Red Star Yeast
(800) 4-CELIAC; (800) 423-5422
carol.stevens@ufoods.com
www.redstaryeast.com

Rice Innovations Inc.
See Pastariso

Road's End Organics
120 Pleasant Street, Suite E-1
Morrisville, VT 05661
(877) CHREESE; (802) 888-2646 (Fax)
roadsend@together.net
www.chreese.com

Safeway (Vons) Stores
P.O. Box 523
Clackamas, OR 92015
(503) 657-6279; (503) 557-4008 (Fax)
www.safeway.com

San-J International, Inc.
2880 Sprouse Drive
Richmond, VA 23231
(804) 226-8333; (800) 446-5500;
(804) 226-8383 (Fax)
sales@san-j.com
www.san-j.com

Sargento Products
800-CHEESES; (800) 558-5802
www.sargento.com

Schillings Spices
See McCormick

Signature Brands
See Betty Crocker

Spangler Candy Company
400 N. Portland Street
P.O. Box 71
Bryan, OH 43506-0071
(419) 636-4221; (800) 653-8638;
(419) 636-3695
Spangler@bright.net
www.spanglercandy.com

Special Foods
9207 Shotgun Court
Springfield, VA 22153
(703) 644-0991; (703) 644-1006 (Fax)
www.specialfoods.com

Stagg
P.O. Box 800
Austin, MN
(800) 611-9778
staggchili@usmpagency.com
www.staggchili.com

Starkist Seafood Co.
One Riverfront Place
Newport, KY 41071
(800) 252-1587
www.starkist.com

Sun-Bird (Williams Foods, Inc.)
13301 West 99th Street
Lenexa, KS 66215
(800) 255-6736
www.hy-vee-stores.com/venders/Williams/
   oriental.htm

Sylvan Border Farm Gluten-Free Products
Mendocino Gluten-Free Products, Inc.
P.O. Box 277
Willits, CA 95490
(800) 297-5399; (707) 459-1834 (Fax)
http://catalog.com/mendo/gcm/sylvan.html

Tamarind Tree, Ltd. (Annie's Homegrown)
P.O. Box 128
Hampton, CT 06247
(781) 224-9639; (800) HFC-TREE;
(781) 224-9728 (Fax)
www.tamtree.com

Tinkyada
120 Melford Drive, Unit 8
Scarborough, Ontario, Canada
M1B 2X5
(416) 609-0016; (416) 609-1316 (Fax)
www.tinkyada.com

Tom's of Maine
P.O. Box 710
Kennebunk, ME 04043
(207) 985-2944; (800) 775-2388;
(207) 985-2196 (Fax)
www.tomsofmaine.com

Tootsie Roll Industries, Inc.
7401 South Cicero
Chicago, IL 60629
(773) 838-3400; (800) 877-7655
www.tootsie.com

Trader Joe's
P.O. Box 3270
South Pasadena, CA 91031
(626) 441-2024; (626) 441-9573 (Fax)
www.traderjoes.com

Tyson Foods, Inc.
P.O. Box 2020
Springdale, AR 72765-2020
(501) 290-4000; (800) 643-3410;
(800) 233-6332
comments@tyson.com
www.tyson.com

U.S. Mills, Inc.
200 Reservoir Street
Needham, MA 02494
(781) 444-0440

Van's International Foods
20318 Gramercy Place
Torrance, CA 90501
(310) 320-8611
www.vansintl.com

Vons (Safeway) Stores
(800) 955-8667
www.vons.com

Whole Foods Market, Inc.
Research and Support Team
601 N. Lamar, Ste. 300
Austin, TX 78703
(512) 477-4455
rs.team@wholefoods.com
www.wholefoodsmarket.com

Williams Foods, Inc.
13301 West 99th Street
Lenexa, KS 66215
(800) 255-6736
www.williamsfoods.com

Wishbone (Lipton)
Consumer Service Department
800 Sylvan Avenue
Englewood Cliffs, NJ 07632
(800) 697-7897
comments.wish-boneusa@unilever.com
www.wish-bone.com

Pharmaceutical Companies and Drug Information

Contact information for pharmaceutical companies is included here so you can check the gluten-free status of over-the-counter and prescription drugs your child uses.

Abbott Laboratories
200 Abbott Park Road
Abbott Park, IL 60064
(847) 937-6100; (800) 441-4987;
(847) 937-9826 (Fax)
www.abbott.com

AstraZeneca LP
725 Chesterbrook Blvd.
Wayne, PA 19087
(610) 695-1000; (800) 237-8898
www.usa.zeneca.com

Barr Labs
2 Quaker Road
Pomona, NY 10970
(800) 222-4043; (914)353-4530 (Fax)
www.barrlabs.com/home.html

Drug Company Phone Numbers
www.needymeds.com/companies.html

Gluten-Free Drug and Food Database
Operator: Clan Thompson
951 Main Street
Stoneham, ME 04231
(207) 928-3303
observer@nxi.com
www.clanthompson.com

Johnson & Johnson
750 Camp Hill Road
Fort Washington, PA 19034
(800) 469-5268; (215) 273-4070 (Fax)
www.jnj.com

Ortho-McNeil Pharmaceutical
1000 U.S. Route 202
P.O. Box 300
Raritan, NJ 08869
(800) 682-6532
www.ortho-mcneil.com

Parke Davis/Warner Lambert (Pfizer)
Patient Assistance Program
P.O. Box 1058
Somerville, NJ 08876
(908) 725-1247; (800) 223-0432;
(908) 707-9544 (Fax)
www.warner-lambert.com; www.pfizer.com

Pfizer, Inc.
Pfizer Prescription Assistance
P.O. Box 25457
Alexandria, VA
(800) 646-4455; (800) 438-1985
www.pfizer.com

Pharmacia & Upjohn
RxMAP
P.O. Box 29043
Phoenix, AZ 85038
(888) 691-6813; (602) 314-7163 (Fax)
ptinfo@pnu.com
www.pnu.com

Proctor & Gamble Pharmaceuticals
Patient Assistance Program
17 Eaton Ave.
Morwich, NY 13815
(800) 448-4878; (800) 836-0658;
(800) 283-8915
atyourservice.im@pg.com
www.pg.com/main.jhtml

Stokes Pharmacy
"Celiac Sprue, A Guide Through the
   Medicine Cabinet"
639 Stokes Road
Medford, NJ 08055
(800) 754-5222; (800) 440-5899 (Fax)
pharmacist@stokesrx.com
www.stokesrx.com

Whitehall-Robins Healthcare
P.O. Box 16609
Richmond, VA 23261-6609
(800) 322-3129; (804) 652-6400 (Fax)
www.healthfront.com

Restaurants and Fast-Food Chains

Applebee's International Restaurant
4551 W. 107th Street, Suite 100
Overland Park, KS 66207
(913) 967-4000; (800) 354-7363 x. 4087;
(913) 967-8984
www.applebees.com

Baskin-Robbins
600 North Brand Blvd., 6th Floor
Glendale, CA 91203
(818) 956-0031; (800) 331-0031;
(818) 548-1283 (Fax)
www.baskinrobbins.com

Burger King
Corporation Consumer Relations
17777 Old Cutler Road
Miami, FL 33157
(305) 378-3535; (305) 378-7011
www.burgerking.com

Chevy's
2000 Powell Street, Suite 200
Emeryville, CA 94608
(800) 4-Chevys; (510) 768-1330 (Fax)
www.chevys.com

Dairy Queen/Orange Julius
7505 Metro Blvd.
P.O. Box 39286
Edina, MN 55439
(952) 830-0200; (952) 830-0480 (Fax)
www.dairyqueen.com

Denny's
203 East Main Street
Box 3-6-9
Spartanburg, SC 29319
(800) 733-6697
tell_us@advantica-dine.com
www.dennys.com

El Pollo Loco
3333 Michelson Drive, Suite 550
Irvine, CA 92612
(949) 399-2000
www.elpolloloco.com

In-N-Out Burgers
4199 Campus Drive, 9th Floor
Irvine, CA 92612
(800) 786-1000
www.in-n-out.com

Jack-in-the-Box
9330 Balboa Avenue
San Diego, CA 92123-1516
(858) 571-2121; (800) 955-5225
www.jackinthebox.com

McDonald's
999 Waterside Drive, Suite 2300
Norfolk, VA 23510
(757) 626-1900; (757) 640-3615 (Fax)
www.mcdonalds.com

Outback Steakhouse
2202 N.W. Shore Blvd.
Tampa, FL 33607
(813) 282-1225; (813) 282-1209 (Fax)
www.outbacksteakhouse.com

Rubio's Baja Grill (Fish Tacos)
Rubio's Restaurants, Inc.
1902 Wright Place, Suite 300
Carlsbad, CA 92008
(760) 929-TACO; (800) 354-4199;
(760) 929-8203 (Fax)
www.rubios.com

Taco Bell
Consumer Affairs
17901 Von Karman
Irvine, CA 92614-6221
(800) 822-6235
www.tacobell.com

TCBY Yogurt
2855 Cottonwood Parkway, Suite 400
Salt Lake City, UT 84121-7050
(800) 323-1156; (800) 688-8229
consumer@tcby.com
www.tcby.com

Tony Roma's
9304 Forest Lane, Suite 2000
Dallas, TX 75243
(800) 286-7662; (214) 343-2680 (Fax)
www.tonyromas.com

Wendy's International, Inc.
Wendy's Customer Service
4288 W. Dublin-Granville Road
Dublin, OH 43017
(614) 764-3100; (800) 82-WENDY
www.wendys.com/index0.html

Publications
Newsletters and Magazines
Many of the national support groups listed above also have subscription publications or distribute periodicals to members.

Bob & Ruth's Gluten-Free Dining and Travel Club
(Newsletter)
22 Breton Hill Road
Baltimore, MD 21208
(410) 486-0292
bobolevy@erols.com

The Gluten-Free Baker Newsletter
361 Cherrywood Drive
Fairborn, OH 45324-4012
(937) 878-3221
thebaker@concentric.net

Gluten-Free Living
Contact: Ann Whelan
P.O. Box 105
Hastings-on-Hudson, NY 10706
(914) 969-2018
gfliving@aol.com

The Gut Reaction
(Gluten-Free Pantry)
(800) 291-8386
pantry@glutenfree.com
www.glutenfree.com

Sully's Living Without
P.O. Box 132
Clarendon Hills, IL 60514-0132
(630) 415-3378
www.livingwithout.com

Cookbooks and Online Recipes

Adler, Kief. *Beyond the Staff of Life.* Happy Camp, CA: Naturegraph Publishers, 1980.

Celiac Sprue Association (P.O. Box 31700, Omaha, NE 68131-0700; (402) 558-0600; (402) 558-1347 (Fax); celiacs@csaceliacs.org). Publications available include: "Best Recipes from Celiacs;" "Easy, Successful Gluten-Free Recipes;" "Gluten-Free International Recipes;" "Holiday Menus;" "Microwave Recipes."

Dumke, Nicolette. *Easy Breadmaking for Special Diets: Wheat-Free, Milk- And Lactose-Free, Egg-Free, Gluten-Free, Yeast-Free, Sugar-Free, Low Fat, High To Low Fiber.* Louisville, CO: Allergy Adapt (1877 Polk Ave., Louisville, CO 80027; www.food-allergy.org).

Fenster, Carol. *Special Diet Celebrations: No Wheat, Gluten, Dairy, or Eggs.*
Littleton, CO: Savory Palate (8174 S. Holly, PMB 404, Littleton, CO 80122-4004; 800-741-5418;
www.savorypalate.com), 1999.

Fenster, Carole. *Special Diet Solutions: Healthy Cooking without Wheat, Gluten, Dairy, Eggs, Yeast, or
Refined Sugar.* Littleton, CO: Savory Palate (8174 S. Holly, PMB 404, Littleton, CO 80122-4004; 800-
741-5418; www.savorypalate.com), 1997.

Fenster, Carol. *Wheat-Free Recipes and Menus: Delicious Dining without Wheat or Gluten.* Littleton, CO:
Savory Palate (8174 S. Holly, PMB 404, Littleton, CO 80122-4004; 800-741-5418;
www.savorypalate.com),1997.

Gardyne, Allan. *Best Gluten-Free Recipes.* (Recipes can be downloaded for free from website at
www.ozemail.com.au/~coeliac/index.html or write for information to Allan Gardyne, Lot 12 Espla-
nade, Tuan, Queensland, Australia 4650.)

Gioannini, Marilyn. *The Complete Food Allergy Cookbook: The Foods You've Always Loved Without the
Ingredients You Can't Have!* Rocklin, CA: Prima, 1997.

Gluten Free/Casein Free Recipes. Available online at: http://gfcfrecipes.tripod.com

Gluten-Free Recipes and Cooking Tips from the Celiac Disease and Gluten-Free Diet Support Page.
Available online at: www.gluten-free.com/recipes.html

Hagman, Bette. *The Gluten-Free Gourmet Bakes Bread: More Than 200 Wheat-Free Recipes.* New York,
NY: Henry Holt & Company, 2000.

Hagman, Bette. *The Gluten-Free Gourmet Cooks Fast and Healthy: Wheat-Free Recipes With Less Fuss and
Less Fat.* New York, NY: Henry Holt & Company, 2000.

Hagman, Bette. *The Gluten-Free Gourmet: Living Well without Wheat.* 2nd Edition. New York NY: Henry
Holt & Company, 1990.

Hagman, Bette. *More from the Gluten-Free Gourmet: Delicious Dining without Wheat.* New York, NY:
Henry Holt & Company, 2000.

Hills, Hilda C. *Good Food, Gluten Free.* Los Angeles, CA: Keats Publishing, 1976.

Hillson, Beth. *Gluten-Free Pantry Companion: Great Recipes for a Wheat-Free/Gluten-Free Kitchen.*
Glastonbury, CT: Gluten-Free Pantry (800-291-8386; pantry@glutenfree.com; www.glutenfree.com).

Meyer, Elisa. *Feeding Your Allergic Child: Happy Food for Happy Kids: 75 Proven Recipes Free of Wheat,
Dairy, Corn, and Eggs for the Millions of Miserable Children.* New York, NY: St. Martin's Press, 1997.

Sarros, Connie. *Wheat-Free, Gluten-Free Dessert Cookbook.* (Order from 3270 Camden Rue, Cuyahoga
Falls, OH 44223; 330-929-1651; gfcookbook@hotmail.com; www.wsff.com/gfcookbook.)

The Searchable Online Archive of Recipes (SOAR). *Gluten Free Recipes.* Available online from:
http://soar.berkeley.edu/recipes/gluten-free

Publications on Celiac Disease and Food Allergies

Celiac Sprue Association (P.O. Box 31700, Omaha, NE 68131-0700; (402) 558-0600; (402) 558-1347
(Fax); celiacs@csaceliacs.org). Publications available include: "Best of Lifeline" and "For Newly
Diagnosed Celiacs."

Gottschall, Elaine. Breaking the Vicious Cycle: Intestinal Health through Diet. Kirkton, Ontario: Kirkton Press, 1994.

Lowell, Jax Peters. *Against the Grain: The Slightly Eccentric Guide to Living Well Without Gluten or Wheat.* New York, NY: Henry Holt & Company, 1996.

National Digestive Diseases Information Clearinghouse (2 Information Way, Bethesda, MD 20892-3570; 301-654-3810; www.niddk.nih.gov). Publications that can be ordered free of charge or viewed online include: "Celiac Disease" and "Lactose Intolerance."

Philpott, William, and Dwight Kalita. *Brain Allergies: The Psychonutrient and Magnetic Connections.* Lincolnwood, IL: NTC/Contemporary Publishing Company, 2000.

Rapp, Doris. *Allergies and Your Family.* Buffalo, NY: Practical Allergy Research Foundation (P.O. Box 60, Buffalo, NY 14223; 716-875-0398), 1980.

Rapp, Doris. *The Impossible Child in School—At Home: A Guide for Caring Teachers and Parents.* Buffalo, NY: Practical Allergy Research Foundation (P.O. Box 60, Buffalo, NY 14223; 716-875-0398), 1989.

Wark, Wendy. *Living Healthy with Celiac Disease.* (To order, send check or money order in the amount of $12.45 to: AnAffect Marketing, 115 Andover Drive, Exton, PA 19341.)

Whelan, Ann. "A Quick Look at Celiac Disease for Those Who Work with Children." (Pamphlet available from Gluten-Free Living, P.O. Box 105, Hastings-on-Hudson, NY 10706; 914-969-2018.)

Willingham, Theresa. *The Food Allergy Field Guide: A Lifestyle Manual for Families.* Littleton, CO: Savory Palate (8174 S. Holly, PMB 404, Littleton, CO 80122-4004; 800-741-5418; www.savorypalate.com), 2000.

Other Publications

Anderson, Winifred, Stephen Chitwood, and Deidre Hayden. *Negotiating the Special Education Maze: A Guide for Parents and Teachers.* 3rd Edition. Bethesda, MD: Woodbine House, 1997.

Balch, James, and Phyllis Balch. *Prescription for Nutritional Healing: A Practical A-Z Reference to Drug-Free Remedies Using Vitamins, Minerals, Herbs, and Food Supplements.* Wayne, NJ: Avery Publishing Group, 1998.

Canadian Celiac Association (190 Britannia Road East, Unit #11, Mississauga, Ontario, Canada, L4Z 1W6; (905) 507-6208; (800) 363-7296; (905) 507-4673 (Fax); www.celiac.ca). Publications include: "Dermatitis Herpetiformis;" "Teachers' Information about Celiac Disease;" "A Guide for the Diabetic Celiac."

Lewis, Lisa. *Special Diets for Special Kids.* Arlington, TX: Future Horizons (422 E. Lamar, Suite 106, Arlington, TX 76011; 800-489-0727), 1998.

National Digestive Diseases Information Clearinghouse (2 Information Way, Bethesda, MD 20892-3570; 301-654-3810; www.niddk.nih.gov). Publications that can be ordered free of charge or viewed online include: "Diagnostic Tests;" "Lactose Intolerance;" "Nutrition and Your Health;" "Your Digestive System and How It Works."

Satter, Ellyn. *Child of Mine: Feeding with Love and Good Sense.* 3rd Edition. Palo Alto, CA: Bull Publishing Co., 2000.

Satter, Ellyn. *How to Get Your Kid to Eat but Not Too Much.* Palo Alto, CA: Bull Publishing Co., 1987.

Van Dyke, D.C., Philip Mattheis, Susan Schoon Eberly, and Janet Williams, editors. *Medical and Surgical Care for Children with Down Syndrome: A Guide for Parents.* Bethesda, MD: Woodbine House, 1995.

Glossary

Accommodation—A change made to the school, work, or other environment that will allow an individual with disabilities to succeed.

ADA—*See* Americans with Disabilities Act.

ADD—*See* Attention Deficit Disorder.

ADHD—*See* Attention Deficit Hyperactive Disorder.

AGA—*See* Antigliadin Antibody.

Allergen—A substance that instigates an allergic reaction. *See also* Allergy; Histamine.

Allergy—A hypersensitivity or intolerance to a condition or substance (allergen) that spawns an adverse physiological reaction. See Histamine; Immunoglobulin E.

Americans with Disabilities Act (ADA)—The federal law that prohibits *discrimination* against people with *disabilities* in employment, public accommodations, and access to public facilities.

Amino Acid – One of the twenty-five organic acids that link together to form the proteins necessary for life.

Anemia—A condition in which the level of hemoglobin in the blood is too low. Often resulting from the *malabsorption* of iron, this condition is characterized by weakness, lethargy, and overall fatigue.

Anencephaly—A birth defect, possibly resulting from a *folic acid* deficiency during pregnancy, characterized by an absence of all but the most primitive parts of the brain, spinal cord, and skull.

Anesthesiologist—A specialist who administers anesthesia, or medication that causes loss of sensation. Anesthesiologists are responsible for monitoring blood loss and vital signs, as well as pain management in sedated patients undergoing surgery. *See also* Conscious Sedation; Unconscious Sedation.

Antibody—A *protein* produced by the body that attaches to and kills antigens that threaten the body.

Antiendomysial Antibody (EmA)—One of the *antibodies* that a person with *celiac disease* produces when *gluten* is ingested. This antibody responds specifically to substances "attacking" the *endomysium*. It is one of the most important antibodies used for diagnosing celiac disease or detecting the presence of gluten in the diet.

Antigen—Invading organisms such as bacteria, viruses, fungi, or parasites that threaten the body. *See also* Antibody.

Antigliadin Antibody (AGA)—One of the *antibodies* that a person with *celiac disease* produces when *gluten* is ingested. Used for diagnosing celiac disease or detecting the presence of gluten in the diet.

Antihistamine—Medication used to counteract the effects of a *histamine*.

Antireticulin Antibody (ARA)—One of the *antibodies* that a person with *celiac disease* produces when gluten is ingested. Used for diagnosing celiac disease or detecting the presence of gluten in the diet.

ARA—*See* Antireticulin Antibody.

Asymptomatic—Showing few or no *symptoms* of a condition.

Asymptomatic Celiac Disease—Having celiac disease, but showing few or no *symptoms* of it. Many people with celiac disease are asymptomatic.

Atrophy—A wasting away; a diminution in the size of a *cell*, tissue, organ, or part.

Attention Deficit Disorder (ADD)—A condition characterized by inattention and distractibility, but not the hyperactivity seen in *Attention Deficit Hyperactivity Disorder.*

Attention Deficit Hyperactivity Disorder (ADHD)—A condition characterized by distractibility, restlessness, short attention span, impulsivity, and hyperactivity. *See also* Attention Deficit Disorder.

Autoimmune Disorder—The general term for a disorder in which the body's *immune system* produces *antibodies* against itself, the mistaken attack resulting in tissue damage. *Celiac disease* is an autoimmune disorder.

B-cell—A *lymphocyte*, or type of *white blood cell*, of the *immune system* responsible for making *antibodies*. *Allergens* are detected by B-cells in the blood. *See also* T-cell.

Biopsy—A procedure involving the removal of living tissue from the body to examine microscopically for the purpose of diagnosing disease.

"Bleed" Test—A procedure in which the finger is pricked with a needle and blood is squeezed out until the body naturally stops the flow.

B.R.A.T. Diet—Diet consisting of bananas, rice, apples, and dry toast, commonly recommended by pediatricians for children with diarrhea.

Calcium—An element taken in through the diet that is essential for a variety of bodily functions, such as neurotransmission, muscle contraction, and proper heart function. Commonly found in dairy products.

CD—*See* Celiac Disease.

Celiac Disease (CD)—A *genetic autoimmune disorder* in which *gluten intolerance* leads to damage to the lining of the *small intestine*. The incidence is estimated at approximately 1 in 150 to 1 in 250 people worldwide. Also known as *coeliac disease, gluten-sensitive enteropathy*, and *nontropical sprue*.

Cell—The smallest unit of a living organism; the basic structure for tissues and organs.

Central Nervous System—Made up of the brain and spinal cord, this system is responsible for controlling what we think and do.

Chronic Diarrhea—*Ongoing, recurrent* diarrhea.

Chronic Fatigue Syndrome—A condition of prolonged and severe tiredness or weariness (fatigue) that is not relieved by rest and is not directly caused by other conditions.

Coeliac Disease—Alternate spelling of *celiac disease.*

Compensated-Latent Disease—A form of *celiac disease* in which the condition is present, but not visible or active.

Conscious Sedation—Light sedation during which the patient retains airway reflexes and can respond when spoken to. *See also* Anesthesiologist; Unconscious Sedation.

Constipation—Condition in which stools are excessively firm and difficult to excrete during infrequent bowel movements.

Crohn's Disease—An inflammatory bowel disease characterized by scarring of the small intestine and/or colon due to chronic inflammation of the digestive tract. Characterized by diarrhea, abdominal pain, and sometimes blood in the stool.

Dermatitis Herpetiformis (DH)—A disorder, closely related to celiac disease, caused by intolerance to gluten and characterized by external manifestations (rash) as well as damage to the small intestine.

DH—*See* Dermatitis Herpetiformis.

Diabetes – An autoimmune disease characterized by excessive urination and excessive thirst. There are two types: diabetes insipidus is caused by a pituitary deficiency; diabetes mellitus involves an insulin deficiency.

Diarrhea—Loose stools during excessively frequent bowel movements. *See also* Chronic Diarrhea.

Disability—A term used to describe a delay in physical and/or cognitive development. The older term "handicap" is also sometimes used.

Discrimination—Showing favor toward one person, race, or group and prejudice toward another.

Distended—Swollen due to pressure within. A distended abdomen is a common *symptom* of *celiac disease*.

Dominant Trait—A characteristic or condition a child *inherits* because a dominant *gene* for that trait overrides any recessive gene it has been paired with. *See also* Recessive Trait.

EmA—*See* Antiendomysial Antibody.

Endomysial—Involving the *endomysium*.

Endomysium—A sheath of connective tissue that surrounds muscle fibers. In people with *celiac disease*, the *antiendomysial antibody* responds specifically to substances "attacking" the endomysium in the *intestine*.

Endoscope—A narrow, flexible tube inserted into the body when performing an *endoscopy*. The endoscope is lighted and usually has a small clipper that can remove tissue samples.

Endoscopy—A procedure in which an *endoscope* is inserted into a body cavity for visual examination. For the purpose of diagnosing *celiac disease*, the endoscope is threaded through the mouth to the *small intestine*, where a doctor removes tissue samples that are later sent to a lab for *biopsy*.

Enzyme—A *protein* that speeds up a chemical change in the body, such as in the digestion of foods.

Epilepsy—A condition characterized by recurrent seizures (muscle contractions or changes in consciousness) that are caused by abnormal electrical activity in the brain.

Failure to Thrive—Describes a condition in which a child experiences below-average weight gain or below-average increase in height.

False Negative—A test result that incorrectly indicates no disease.

Fatty Stool Test—Used to confirm the presence of *celiac disease*, a stool is examined for high fat content indicated by buoyancy. *See also* Steatorrhea.

Folic Acid – The synthetic form of folate, a B vitamin found naturally in many foods and important for the formation of red and white blood cells.

"Free Appropriate Public Education"—The right, under *IDEA,* of every child with *disabilities* to an education provided at public expense that is appropriate to his or her developmental strengths and needs.

Gastroenterologist—A physician specializing in medical problems associated with the digestive system; qualified to diagnose and supervise the treatment of *celiac disease*.

Gastrointestinal—Relating to the stomach and *intestines*.

Gastrointestinal Distress—The experience of cramping, bloating, gas, or *diarrhea*.

Gene—The basic unit of heredity, located at specific points on chromosomes, made up of DNA and *protein*.

Genetic—Inherited.

"Genetic Fingerprint"- *See* Human Leukocyte Antigen.

GF—*See* Gluten-Free.

Gliadin – The part of the protein in gluten-containing grains that is soluble in alcohol; the *promaline* portion of the *gluten molecule.* The type of reaction an individual with *celiac disease* experiences may be determined by the amount of gliadin in a given food.

Glutelin—A simple protein found in the seeds of cereal grains; a component of gluten. *See also* Promaline.

Gluten—A protein found in wheat, rye, barley, and oats.

Gluten Antibody Blood Test—*See* Serum Antibody Test.

Gluten-Free (GF) – Containing no *gluten*.

Gluten Intolerance—An inability to properly digest foods containing *gluten*.

Gluten-Sensitive Enteropathy (GSE)—Another name for *celiac disease*.

GSE—*See* Gluten-Sensitive Enteropathy.

Gut—An *intestine*; a bowel; the whole alimentary canal (from mouth to anus).

Hemorrhage—Heavy bleeding from a blood vessel.

Histamine—The chemical compound that causes the disagreeable *symptoms* of an allergic reaction. *See also* Allergen; Allergy; Antihistamine.

HLA—*See* Human Leukocyte Antigen.

Human Leukocyte Antigen (HLA)—A *protein* that protrudes from the surface of a person's *cells*. The HLAs, which make up the "genetic fingerprint," allow the *immune* cells in the body to recognize things that belong specifically to that person.

IBS—*See* Irritable Bowel Syndrome.

IDEA—*See* Individuals with Disablilities Education Act.

IEP—*See* Individualized Education Program.

IgA—*See* Immunoglobulin A.

IgE—*See* Immunoglobulin E.

IgG—*See* Immunoglobulin G.

Immune System—The complicated network of molecules that produce antibodies, which eliminate infections caused by bacteria, viruses, and invading microbes, defending the body against disease.

Immunoglobulin A (IgA)—Present in the secretions of the body's mucous membranes, this is one of the *antibodies* that a person with *celiac disease* produces when *gluten* is ingested. Used for diagnosing celiac disease or detecting the presence of gluten in the diet. *See also* Antigliadin Antibody.

Immunoglobulin E (IgE)—One of the *antibodies* produced in response to an *allergen* that a person with *celiac disease* makes when *gluten* is ingested. Used for diagnosing celiac disease or detecting the presence of gluten in the diet.

Immunoglobulin G (IgG)—The primary type of *antibody* that responds to invading organisms in the body. It is one of the antibodies that a person with *celiac disease* produces when *gluten* is ingested. Used for diagnosing celiac disease or detecting the presence of gluten in the diet. *See also* Antigliadin Antibody.

Individualized Education Program (IEP)—The written plan that specifies the services the local education agency has agreed to provide a child with *disabilities* who is eligible under *IDEA*; for children ages three to twenty-one.

Individuals with Disabilities Education Act (IDEA)—A federal law originally passed in 1975 and subsequently amended that requires states to provide a *"free appropriate public education* in the least restrictive environment" to children with *disabilities*.

Infertility—The inability to conceive offspring.

Inherited – Relating to traits, such as eye and hair color or certain conditions, passed through *genes* from one generation to another. Used synonymously with *genetic*.

Intestine—The passageway from the stomach to the anus, consisting of the large and *small intestines*, through which food travels and is digested.

Irritable Bowel Syndrome (IBS)—A functional bowel disorder characterized by recurrent cramping, abdominal pain, and *diarrhea*.

Lactase—An *enzyme* produced in the *small intestine* that breaks *lactose* into two simpler sugars, thereby helping the body to digest lactose.

Lactose—A sugar found in dairy products that can cause an allergic reaction. *See also* Allergy; Lactase; Lactose Intolerance.

Lactose Intolerance—An inability to tolerate *lactose,* which can result in *gastrointestinal distress* Sometimes caused by an interruption in the production of *lactase.* Common in people with untreated celiac disease.

Latent—Present but inactive.

Lupus—An a*utoimmune disorder* in which the body develops *antibodies* against the DNA of its own *cells,* resulting in abnormalities of blood vessels and connective tissue.

Lymphocyte—A *white blood cell* of the *immune system,* lymphocytes are divided into two major classes: *B-cells* and *T-cells.*

Lymphoma—Encompassing a variety of cancers of the lymphatic system, lymphoma is characterized by the uncontrollable multiplication of lymph cells resulting in symptoms such as swelling of the lymph nodes, itching, fatigue, weight-loss, and fever. People with *celiac disease* are 40 to 100 times more likely to develop intestinal lymphoma than those unaffected.

Malabsorption—Inefficient absorption of nutrients from food as it passes from the mouth through the esophagus, stomach, and *intestines* to the anus. Results in *malnourishment.*

Malnourishment—The state of being improperly nourished or sustained by the substances necessary for life and growth.

Miscarriage—A spontaneous end of pregnancy before the fetus has developed sufficiently to survive outside the womb.

Molecule—The smallest particle of an element or compound that can exist in the free state and still maintain its recognizable characteristics.

Mucosal Damage—Injury to the mucous membrane, or lining, of body cavities.

Multigenetic—Describes a condition in which several *genes,* perhaps each having different strengths of expression, are involved in contributing to a specific trait. *Celiac disease* is believed to be multigenetic. *See also* Dominant Trait; Recessive Trait.

Negative Predictive Value—The probability of no disease in a patient with a negative test result. *See also* Positive Predictive Value.

Nontropical Sprue—Another name for *celiac disease.*

Osteomalacia—A condition caused by vitamin D deficiency, leading to the loss of calcium from bones. This, in turn, can result in weakened bones or fractures. The same condition in children is called rickets.

Osteoporosis—A reduction in the amount of bone mass, so that fractures can occur after minimal trauma.

Pediatric Gastroenterologist (Pediatric G.I.)—A *gastroenterologist* whose patients are children.

Pediatric G.I.—*See* Pediatric Gastroenterologist.

Phlebotomist—A professional who draws blood using a needle and tourniquet.

Positive Predictive Value—The probability of disease in a patient with a positive test result. *See also* Negative Predictive Value.

Prolamine—A simple *protein* found in plants that cannot be dissolved in anything except strong alcohol solutions. It is an important component of *gluten*. Also spelled prolamin. *See also* Gliadin; Glutelin.

Protein—An organic compound, made up of linked *amino acids,* necessary for life.

Raynaud Syndrome – A condition in which the small arteries in the fingers and toes have spasms, resulting in pale or patchy skin and numbness or tingling.

Recessive Trait—A characteristic or condition that is inherited only when the gene for that trait is transmitted to the offspring by both parents. *See also* Dominant Trait.

Rehabilitation Act of 1973—*Section 504* of this federal law prohibits *discrimination* against individuals with *disabilities* in federally funded programs.

Reticulin—Constituent *protein* of reticular fibers: collagen type III.

Rickets—A childhood disease caused by a *vitamin D* deficiency. Characterized by abnormalities in the shape and structure of bones, body tenderness, sweating of the head, and an enlarged liver and spleen. *See also* Osteomalacia.

Schizophrenia—A mental disorder characterized by disturbances in form and content of thought, mood, sense of self and relationship to the outside world, and behavior.

Section 504—*See* Rehabilitation Act of 1973.

Sensitivity—The probability of a positive test result in a patient with disease. *See also* Specificity.

Serological Test—A blood test.

Serum Antibody Test—A blood test that detects the presence of antibodies to a particular antigen. In celiac disease, the test can provide evidence of gluten in the body. Also known as Gluten Antibody Blood Test.

Small Intestine—Extending from the stomach to the large *intestine*, the small intestine is composed of three sections: duodenum, jejunum, and ileum. All are involved in the absorption of nutrients. In celiac disease, the duodenum is first to be affected.

Specificity—The probability of a negative test result in a patient without disease. *See also* Sensitivity.

Spina Bifida—A condition in which a part of the spinal column fails to close completely before birth, resulting in varying degrees of physical impairment and paralysis.

Steatorrhea—A condition, characterized by foul, frothy, sometimes floating stools, in which there is an abnormally large amount of fat in the stool; usually the result of poor absorption in the *small intestine* as in *celiac disease*. *See also* Fatty Stool Test.

Symptom—An indication of a disease or disorder that is noticed by a patient and can help in reaching a diagnosis.

T-cell—A critical *lymphocyte,* or type of *white blood cell*, of the *immune system* that aids in destroying infected *cells* and coordinates the overall immune response.

Thyroid Disease—A disease of the thyroid gland, which secretes hormones important for controlling body metabolism. "Hypothyroid" describes an underactive thyroid gland; "hyperthyroid" describes an overactive thyroid gland.

Tissue Transglutaminase (tTG) – A blood *test* that measures *EmA-IgA* levels. Very specific to detecting the presence of *antibodies* released by people with *celiac disease* when *gluten* is ingested.

tTG—*See* Tissue Transglutaminase.

Unconscious Sedation—Sedation in which the patient is completely "asleep" during surgery. *See also* Anesthesiologist; Conscious Sedation.

Villi—Small hair-like projections on certain mucous membranes in the body that secrete mucus and absorb nutrients from digested food. People with celiac disease can become *malnourished* and dehydrated if the villi in the intestine are damaged by gluten and cannot perform their function.

Vitamin D—The "sunshine vitamin" produced by the body when exposed to UV light. Plays an important role in *calcium* and phosphorus metabolism. *See also* Osteomalacia; Rickets.

White Blood Cell—One of three types of blood cells. They protect the body by destroying harmful or foreign substances such as bacteria, viruses, and fungi.

Zonulin—Recently discovered in high levels in individuals with *celiac disease*, this *protein* opens the spaces between *cells*, allowing some substances to pass though, while preventing harmful bacteria and toxins from entering.